❦

'No one ever stayed slim for very long just

because of a diet.'

Paulo Coelho author of The Witch of Portobello

This opening gambit from the master writer Paulo Coelho, is what is at the heart of this book, True Slimness, which I warmly dedicate to my mother Eileen and my breathwork coach Sue Lawson who have both moved on to experience life in the non-physical realms.

❦

Table of Contents

Introduction

DISCLAIMER: The information in this book is for information purposes and a form of sharing my own direct experience in natural permanent weight loss. It is intended to complement not substitute medical advice.

INTRODUCTION

To date, I've had over twenty years of natural permanent slimness. It started the day I gave up dieting, and started to *feel my feelings* instead of eating when full because of them. If I can do it, you can too. So read on, for I know that these forty, True Slimness, weight loss principles can empower you to alter and change your eating habits to those of a naturally slim person, and in so doing, you can, and will, get slim and stay slim for good.

The day-to-day reality of being a recovered compulsive eater is something I would like everyone, who has ever struggled with their weight, to experience. This freedom from excess weight, this freedom from obsession with food, size and shape, is something that I'd striven for, for years, in the wrestling match of emotions, self-image and self-worth, until finally, I overcame it.

So, it is from my own direct experience that I write this book – True Slimness. In it, I share with you what worked for me, knowing it can be a roadmap for you, to discover true, and lasting, slimness.

Please note: This weight loss method is suitable for both men and women, however, I predominately use the female pronoun because my work has 99% been with women. I also use the female pronoun for consistency, and have found it interesting to notice, that the word 'woman' contains the word 'man – wo(man), and the word 'she' contains the word 'he' – s(he). So both the feminine and the masculine are represented beautifully.

What is an excess amount of food?

Excess food causes excess weight. Now this simple truth begs the all-important question – What is an excess amount of food?

Well, after a lifetime of finishing everything on our plates, or restricting our food intake, we might have become either unable to contact, or completely ignoring of our hunger and fullness sensations, and these are the very sensations that will tell you when to eat, *and,* how much to eat.

The fullness sensation, when acted upon appropriately by 'stopping when physically full,' allows the food already in the stomach to be digested, absorbed, converted into energy, and used to renew this intricate, miraculous organism known as the human body. Let us no longer ignore or dismiss as unimportant, these subtle, inner, hunger and fullness sensations. Instead, let us consider the hunger and fullness sensations as messages of inner wisdom, that are guiding us to greater health, natural slimness, and overall well-being.

Your stomach is a bridge if you like, a bridge between you and food; and as all body organs, it has an innate intelligence specific to its task. Now, I appreciate that it might be hard to believe that an internal organ, such as the stomach, has a form of *knowing* or intelligence, but if you think about it, how does the heart *know* how to beat? How do the lungs *know* how, and when, to inhale and exhale? How do the kidneys *know* how to cleanse the blood? They know, and they do it effortlessly, without any conscious effort on our part. So too, the stomach *knows* exactly how much food you need, to fuel, your particular body, and it relays this *knowing* through the fullness sensation. It knows when it needs more fuel, and relates that to us via the hunger sensation. It is this natural, inner knowing that all naturally slim folk automatically trust, and follow. And it is this inner knowing, that I am asking you to reconnect with, trust, and follow, as one of your first steps on your journey towards true, and lasting, slimness. It is this inner knowing, of when you are genuinely physically hungry, and genuinely physically full, that will get you slim, and keep you slim.

In the following, we will discover how to become more aware of it and how to follow it, and thus, get permanently slim because of it. That inner knowing, of when we are hungry, and when we are full, is your guide now.

So, let's begin. The stomach sends us hunger signals when it needs more food, or fuel for the body to function at its best. Fuel, which is turned into the energy that quite literally, keeps us alive. Obviously, if we ignore its, 'stop the inflow of fuel' signal, which comes in the form of the fullness sensation, and give it too much fuel, that extra fuel is what gets turned into fat. Therefore, food eaten whilst ignoring the stomach's fullness sensation, that is, food eaten when physically full, is not all used up as energy or replenishment of tissues and cells, but is stored as fat cells on the body. This means – eating when physically full, is, the direct cause of excess weight.

The innate intelligence of the body is always seeking to establish the body's own natural weight. That natural weight is different for each of us. A six foot four man's natural weight obviously will not be the same as a petit, five foot two, lady. Each body knows what its own natural weight is, and seeks to establish it through the hunger and fullness sensations. Our own natural weight is always slim, not stick insect slim, but, a healthy slimness, a natural slimness, a slimness that can be naturally achieved by stopping eating when physically full.

True Slimness Weight Loss Principle # 1 The fullness sensation tells us when enough is enough concerning our food intake. *Food when full* is excess food, and the direct cause of excess weight.

True Slimness Weight Loss Principle # 2 Listen to, trust and act on the stomach's hunger and fullness sensations.

7

Some women say to me – *But this is far too simple to be the effective solution.*

And my answer is - *Yes it is simple, and we human beings sometimes overlook or dismiss the simple solutions in life. However, many of the most profound things in life are simple, but your own individual complexities do come to the fore as the mystery unravels, and you delve into your emotional reasons, for eating when full.*

Others have asked me – *If it is this simple, why haven't we been doing it already?*

And my answer is – *We were not allowed to do it.*

Let me explain:

As children, when our parents, relatives or teachers told us to 'eat up' even though our stomachs told us we were already physically full, we subtly got the message, that we cannot trust our own natural fullness sensation as the ultimate authority on when to stop eating. We learned that our fullness sensation was not really that important. We learned that the simple truth, of being physically full, was not worthy of our respect. We learned, that the simple sensation of being physically full, was not worth paying attention to, or obeying, and, as a result, we gained weight. We learned the habit of ignoring and disobeying the fullness sensation, we got into the habit of eating when full, and we got fat.

Being physically full, we learned, was simply not a good enough reason to stop eating.

In truth, the hunger and fullness sensations can be listened to and trusted. When we were babies we all automatically recognised and obeyed them. We cried when hungry until the breast or bottle was available, and we stopped suckling when full. And toddlers are famous for pushing away that spoonful of baby food that mother is happily offering, and even if the well-meaning mother does manage to get that spoonful of food in the little mouth, it is promptly spat out! So in tune with their fullness sensations, they intuitively recognise its importance! This is the kind of attitude I'm encouraging you to get back to, hopefully without the crying and spitting.

When we no longer push our children to eat beyond physical fullness, our children's natural trust in their own bodies fullness sensation gets validated. This allows a natural, healthy and enjoyable relationship to food to be established, as nature intended.

☙

Have you ever considered that whoever encouraged you to eat when full, by asking you to finish everything on your plate, was wrong? Well-meaning, well-intentioned, but wrong.

It is true, these well-meaning people, who did their very best, were in fact labouring under a misconception - the misconception that *it is okay to eat when full.* And, the belief, *it is okay to eat when full,* is a fat-creating belief. So, let's here and now, take on a new belief, the belief that it is okay to stop when full. *That* is the ultimate slimness-creating belief. Our actions spring out of our beliefs, so thus empowered, you move forward, into, and keep, with a firm foundation, your slim-self.

My workshop participants invariably point out, that encouragement to eat when full sprang out of genuine scarcity, or fear of there not being enough food. Generations ago, and even in recent times, when lack of food *was a reality* many faced, demanding empty places was literally a survival tactic. I address this issue by stating that hopefully none of us need to adopt such drastic measures, and, even if money is tight and food seems in short supply, I have found in my own experience, that a little careful budgeting, and creativity, is a gentler, and far more effective solution that does <u>not</u> cause anyone to gain weight in the name of shortage. They say old habits die hard. Well, I am not so sure that is true, but die they must, in order for the new, more effective, slim–friendly and life-enhancing habits, patterns and beliefs to emerge and replace them. Nothing likes to die, even that which is no longer serving you well, so there may be a little inner conflict, but that soon dies down as the rewards, of the new habits, and belief that *it is okay to stop when full*, are experienced.

☯

Sometimes it is painful for us, as adults, to realise that our parents are only human and are capable of making mistakes. This realisation, along with uncomfortable feelings, may surface when you are around your parents whilst practising your new habit of stopping when full. (See the Am I hungry? assignment on page 15). Even though you are changing the way you eat, your parents will probably still be employing the old ways. Just being aware, of *how you feel* as you notice their eating patterns, comments, and attitudes, about weight and food, helps.

The good news is, that no matter what sort of misguidance we suffered as children, we can change everything we need to change about our eating habits now, in order to make them slim-friendly eating habits. Let us start here. The simplicity of it *is*, really amazing! When we listen out for our fullness sensations, we automatically *know* what the right amount of food is, for we *feel* physically full. If we feel over-stuffed, then we know we've simply gone beyond that original fullness sensation and run the risk of gaining some weight.

Now, the hunger and fullness sensations are subtle sensations, and it does take a little awareness, and practice, to get back in tune with these silent messages emanating from the stomach, and a willingness to do that goes a long way in helping you establish a strong connection to them. So lets explore why, and how, to pay attention to these inner whispers, that state very clearly, either – 'I'm hungry now', or, 'I'm full now.'

To stop eating when full is natural.

To stop eating when full is the natural mechanism through which the body regulates its own weight.

Both the absorption of any excess fat cells and the maintaining of natural slimness is achieved directly through stopping when full.

Our job now, is to practice it as our new way of eating.

Our job now, is to practice stopping when full.

The amount of food you need, is not always a static thing, and is influenced by several variables. These variables include, how long it's been since you last ate, whether or not you do physical work, or exercise regularly, what amount of energy you have recently expended, and whether or not you overate recently. Miraculously, all of this is taken into consideration by that innate intelligence I spoke about earlier, and the built-in hunger and fullness sensations. It is this built–in, weight-regulating mechanism that I encourage you to trust now, for it can tell you all you need to know, in order to lose weight, and maintain that weight loss regardless of whether you lead an active or sedentary lifestyle.

- For a day spent mostly sitting down, all you need to know about how much to eat, is relayed to you, via your hunger and fullness sensations.

- For a day that you go out on a five-mile walk, all you need to know, about how much to eat, is relayed to you via your hunger and fullness sensations.

- If you carry 7 extra pounds, all you need to know, to lose that weight is relayed to you via your hunger and fullness sensations.

- If you have 70 or more extra pounds to lose, all you need to know, to lose that excess weight, is relayed to you via your hunger and fullness sensations.

- If you are slim, or when you get slim, all you need know, to keep that slimness, is relayed to you, via your hunger and fullness sensations.

So, I trust I have been successful in driving home the point of how all-important these sensations are, in the achieving, and maintaining of weight loss.

True Slimness Weight Loss Principle # 3 Eliminate all eating when physically full.

Now that we wholeheartedly know that it is the eating when we are physically full that causes excess weight, it logically follows that in order to lose the excess weight, we have got to *lose*, or eliminate, the excess eating – the eating when physically full.

Our goal? To stop when full.

It is our goal now, to get to the stage where we are automatically eating when physically hungry, and stopping when physically full, 100% of the time. It may sound simple enough, but to the compulsive eater, it can be as hard as giving up an addiction, for that is exactly what we are doing – giving up an addiction – an addiction to *food when full*.

I say to my clients – 'Turn your ear inwards, and listen to your stomach, not just when it is growling with hunger, but listen out for those subtle sensations of slight hunger. The type of hunger that a sandwich and a cup of coffee would satisfy.'

We also need to be aware of what I call *food fancyings* that tell us – *I would really love a tuna sandwich.* In this way, we are listening to the specific vitamin and mineral needs of our body, for that moment in time. This is why, one day you fancy an orange juice with your lunch (your body is specifically telling you it requires some vitamin C), and the next day you fancy a large bottle of mineral water (a need for hydration). For dinner on Tuesday, you fancy a spicy beanburger and chips, whereas Wednesday, it's soup and garlic bread (garlic is a natural antibiotic, and beans a source of protein). One day, fruit salad is the order of the day, and it's fish and chips the next. Our bodies, truly are, perfect systems, operating with a perfect, physical, inner harmony, which guarantees us, perfect physical health – *if we listen to them and act on their guidance.* The subtle and quiet messages of **when to feed ourselves and what to feed ourselves,** is constantly being relayed to us via our hunger and fullness sensations, and our food fancyings. Whether or not we pick up on, and obey these signals, is up to us. Good health and losing excess weight is guaranteed as we follow their cue.

So why do we eat when full?

'Why do we allow overindulgence to lead to an epidemic of obesity when our cells measure to the molecule how much fuel we consume?' Dr Deepak Chopra

This is a very important question the bestselling author, Dr Deepak Chopra has raised. Why do so many of us eat when full, considering that the body does indeed 'measure to the molecule how much fuel we consume' and has in-built signals (the hunger and fullness sensations) that actually tell us when to start, and when to stop eating, in a constant monitoring of that fuel, in order for us to achieve, and maintain, perfect weight? Why do we override the intelligence that seeks only to help us get slim and stay slim and healthy? Well, the answer is, emotional.

True Slimness Weight Loss Principle # 4 Eating when full suppresses feelings.

Let me endeavour to explain. A woman with an eating disorder can have such a strained relationship to food that she habitually, over-rides, the subtle, inner cues which are telling her whether her stomach is full or empty. She can be so, out of touch, with when she is physically hungry and when she is physically full, that she is stuffing her face when her stomach is screaming at her NO MORE FOOD PLEASE! And when her stomach is saying – *I would like a nice hot bowl of soup* – she refuses to eat. This, is an example of a woman not meeting her body's needs appropriately. This, is pretty much, a self-abusive activity. Consciously or subconsciously, she is indulging in this self-abusive activity in order to suppress her feelings. To eat when physically full is *one* way of dealing with unpleasant or uncomfortable feelings and unresolved emotional issues. Whatever these feelings or issues may be, she is using *food when full* to suppress them. Is that woman you? She certainly used to be me.

This business of suppressing feelings is not always a conscious urge. In other words, when we have the urge to binge, we don't always consciously think – 'I just gotta suppress this anger.' No, we often only have an awareness of the overwhelming urge to eat, even though we know, we are physically full. We feel a binge coming on – we just know that we are gonna eat that chocolate cake, even though we already are, very full. It has an, *out of control,* quality to it, and we may or may not be aware, that what's really driving us to eat when full, is the fact that we are peeved with the next door neighbour, or mad at our spouse, or physically exhausted and in need of a quiet nap.

Question: How do we begin to break out of this inappropriate cycle, which is a very self-abusive way of, not only eating, but of dealing with feelings and emotional issues?

Answer: The following assignment.

This assignment shows us how to unravel the dysfunctional links between eating and feelings, so that we can put both food, and feelings, in their proper place in our day-to-day lives. It incorporates our first, four, True Slimness weight loss principles, and allows all four principles to be operating for maximum benefit. Practice asking yourself often, the key question – **Am I hungry?** And follow through on the guidelines in columns A and B. The first few weeks and months of healing the habit of eating when full, will be spent mastering this simple, yet empowering procedure, which I have named - **Am I hungry?** This, I have found, can be a very rewarding and interesting time.

Every time you think about food or eating, ask yourself – Am I physically hungry? Just before you eat, ask yourself – Am I physically hungry?

A. Yes	B. No
Eat whatever you fancy until physically full. When physically full, stop eating until you are physically hungry again.	This is emotional hunger; you still want to eat even though you are physically full. At this moment it is vital to ask yourself - 1. What feeling is this? 2. Given the fact I feel this way what would I like to do now? 3. If the answer is a healthy one, get busy doing it.

Please note, the **Am I hungry?** assignment is by far the most important assignment in this whole program, for it is practically the whole program condensed. Memorise it, practice it, and practice it some more, until it is automatic. Photocopy it, and paste it to your fridge. Have a copy of it by your bedside, and carry one in your handbag or pocket, to read whenever you have a spare moment.

Do be aware of what your mind comes up with as an *answer* to the question – Given the fact I feel this way what would I like to do now? Make sure the answer is *a healthy alternative to stuffing the feelings down,* and not just another avoidance tactic, such as lighting a fag, a binge on wine, or a compulsive shopping spree, *just to cheer yourself up,* but leaves you in debt. These activities are simply other ways of avoiding, or suppressing, those uncomfortable feelings and emotional issues that have been triggering your episodes of eating when full. It is important to allow yourself to *feel your feelings* and <u>not</u> suppress them. It is very important that **how** you react to, and act on, your feelings, **is** helping you to resolve them. To clarify this point, take a look at the example below:

Example:

I feel like eating and I check in with my stomach, I ask myself –

> **Am I physically hungry?**

> The answer comes – 'No, I am physically full.'

> So, (as outlined in column B) I check in with my feelings by asking –

> **What feeling is this?**

> I realise I'm bored. I then ask myself –

> **Given the fact I feel this way (bored), what would I like to do now?**

> The answer comes – I would like to phone a friend. I look through my phone book and call one of my friends, enjoy a chat and feel satisfied.

This is a simple example of easily meeting your own emotional needs appropriately, and, you have just sidetracked a binge!

I am sure I don't have to remind you that it is not always as simple as this. There could be bigger issues involved. However, the important thing is to become aware of those issues, feel the feelings associated with them, and know that deep within you lies the solution to those issues, no matter how big or small, or how old or painful they may be. Some emotional issues are easy to resolve, and some are not, the main thing, here, is to just *allow a willingness to be open to whatever comes up,* knowing that, in truth, you can handle whatever comes up. Even if some emotional biggies surface, you'll find reserves of strength within you, and ways to move forward before you, that you've never before experienced. Those emergency reserves of strength emerge when we feel weak, or at breaking point, but look at it this way - it is a breaking point for a *breakthrough.* It is, as if we have to break a hard shell of negative consciousness, in order for the new strength and circumstances to evolve, and solutions to be recognised and used. And that is when a really, big, healing takes place, and moves us forward in life freed from an old burden, be it a release from some old, emotional baggage, or a physical improvement in health, finances, or relationships, the evidence will be there, in your life, as a lovely reminder that you went that second mile, and reaped the benefits of refusing to stuff down emotional issues, and allowed yourself to *feel your feelings* rather than *suppress those feelings by eating when full.*

But most of what comes up for us emotionally is easy to deal with, and ways open to us that seem, simple, logical and easy to follow, and sometimes, ways open to us that we never dreamed of as being possible, and thankfully we allow their goodness into our life.

This is an amazing journey that can bring so much big and small positive change into your life. Positive changes that only come as a result of having dealt with, that previously suppressed, emotional stuff.

Remember, you get slim as a direct result of eating when hungry and stopping when full. And stopping when full puts you in the position where your emotional stuff can be felt and dealt with, rather than suppressed.

The mainstream idea is, that you get slim and then your life improves. However, it is more accurate to say that *it is only through feeling and resolving the previously suppressed emotional stuff, that life improves.* The true key, to any improvement in your life, will always lie in feeling and resolving the emotional stuff that you previously stuffed down by eating food when physically full. And the aforementioned **Am I Hungry?** assignment is your basic blueprint for doing just that.

You no longer have to suppress your emotional stuff by eating when full.

You no longer have to ignore and perpetuate your emotional issues by suppressing them by eating when physically full and thus creating another problem – the excess weight.

As we give up 'eating when full' we become women who face up to, and resolve our emotional issues, leaving us free to move forward into the life of our choice. The life of good health, slimness, satisfying work, supportive friendships, fulfilling relationships, enjoyable pastimes and prosperity. This surely is, the life we all aspire to, and can have through self-understanding, self-belief, self-healing and self-effort.

☯

The more we eat when physically hungry and stop when physically full, the more we are *creating a clear channel through which feelings can flow.* We quite literally, are no longer *suppressing* but instead are *experiencing* those old previously suppressed feelings. It is directly through the *experiencing* or *feeling of feelings*, especially uncomfortable ones, that they get healed. Please note: Experiencing and feeling feelings does not necessarily involve acting on them, especially with feelings such as anger. It is vitally important to act appropriately on our feelings, so that they heal, and not just go about dumping them on others. Later in the book we will look at healthy, non-dumping methods, of dealing with feelings such as anger.

☯

It is through the added awareness of how we feel emotionally that our issues are more easily resolved, and once resolved, these emotional issues never again cause us to eat when full, in order to cope with them, for we have indeed found other, more effective ways of coping, through our practice of the **Am I hungry?** guidelines. And, as you continue to, daily practice, the **Am I hungry?** guidelines, you are in the powerful position of not only being able to cope with your feelings and emotional issues in better ways, but you are also, well on the way to resolving permanently, anything, that previously bothered you. The permanent resolving of an emotional issue is always accompanied by life getting better in some way, shape or form, and that alone, surely provides encouragement enough, for *going through,* rather than *suppressing* the less pleasant, of life's emotions.

True Slimness Weight Loss Principle # 5 Addiction is any activity that suppresses feelings. *Eating when full* suppresses feelings, therefore *eating when full* is food addiction.

The following enables you to see what your choices are:

Choice (A) The *stuff my feelings down* way

- I am aware of my emotional issue and I am feeling some uncomfortable feelings – I indulge in food addiction, that is, I eat when physically full thus suppressing my feelings.

- Or, starting off hungry and eating, but continuing to eat long past the time when my stomach has become physically full.

- Or, indulge in another addiction, such as light a cigarette, or have a gin and tonic, or watch too much TV, or spend on a credit card that I can't pay off in one, full, payment.

- As a result of any of the above three activities, the emotional issue remains unresolved and my energy is depleted as it takes a lot of energy to keep a feeling under wraps.

- If I have eaten when full I will gain weight. If I have smoked I will be damaging my lungs. If I drank alcohol, especially in excess, it tends to leave the body in an acidic state, which some say, is the foundation for all ill health.

Choice (B) The *feel my feelings and integrate my feelings* way

- I am aware of my emotional issue and am feeling some uncomfortable feelings – I feel my feelings, this enables them to integrate. I recognise my feelings if possible, for example, anger, fear, boredom, annoyed or impatient.

- I do not eat if I am physically full, even though I may have a strong urge to do so.

- I ask myself – Given the fact I feel this way what would I like to do now?

- Then I do whatever comes to mind as the intuitive answer. If no answer comes to mind, then I am able to simply relax and be aware of, or *allow*, my feelings until they pass. I am feeling my feelings, I am conscious of them passing. I may get ideas of an action or actions to take now, tomorrow or the next day, or a whole plan of action might come to mind as I stay conscious of how I am feeling at this moment in time that I have the urge to eat when full (binge). As in the coming days I follow up on those ideas and take action, the emotional issue gets resolved, and my energy is freed up. I feel energised.

- As I continue to eat when physically hungry and stop when physically full, I am putting my body in the position whereby it can automatically absorb any excess fat. When there is no more excess fat and I continue to eat when physically hungry and stop when physically full, I am in the position whereby my body can maintain that weight loss. Again, both the absorption of excess weight and the maintaining of my slim body is a direct result of eating when physically hungry and stopping when physically full.

Do acknowledge that with past traumas what you are aiming for here is the ability to feel the feelings and deal with the trauma in such a way as to ensure that it no longer has a negative effect on your life today, or has the power to cause you to binge. With a trauma such as the death of a loved one, there is the acknowledgement that, of course, you are never the same after such a loss, and within that you are still able to learn ways of dealing with that loss so that you no longer eat when full because of the pain and grief.

This leads nicely to the obvious importance of finding and using the tools which help you deal with your feelings and unresolved emotional stuff in a healthy appropriate way. The easiest and first of these tools is the aforementioned question - **Given the fact I feel this way what would I like to do now?** This is the question, whose answer, can lead you to the precious, healthy alternative to eating when physically full, the healthy alternative to the binge, the healthy alternative to using *food when full* as an ineffective means of dealing with your feelings, the healthy alternative to the deadly suppression and denial of how we really feel. So, do ask yourself the question - **Given the fact I feel this way what would I like to do now?** whenever you are already physically full, but feel uncomfortable feelings brewing in your awareness, while still craving to eat more, for it will always guide you away from your addiction to food when full, and towards good health. The answer to the question – Given the fact I feel this way, what would I like to do now? – gives you an escape hatch through which to climb out of food addiction and the life sentence of being overweight. It can be viewed as a magic question but it is more accurate to say, it is an *alchemical* question. It quite literally, facilitates the transformation of you, from your fat-self, to your slim-self.

Feeding ourselves emotionally

So, in no uncertain terms, knowing this (what you would like to do at that moment in time, when you are physically full but still crave to eat more) is the means by which you break out of that old, negative pattern of eating when full – the pattern that causes excess weight. And when you put into practice this healthy answer, this healthy alternative (such as phone a friend) you are meeting your own emotional needs appropriately. Thus you can say that you are *feeding yourself emotionally* and are well on the way to reaching your desired destination of true and lasting slimness, for you are dealing directly, and effectively with the root cause of your excess weight –

the unresolved emotional issues and feelings that can drive us to the fridge when full, without even a backward glance.

Please remember when asking – Given the fact I feel this way what would I like to do now? – That it is? – 'What would I *like* to do now? – and not – 'What *should* I do now?'

You *should* be doing the dishes, mowing the lawn, tidying the kitchen, doing the laundry and a thousand and one other things on that infinite to-do list, but what you would *like* to do might be sitting down with a cup of tea and a good book. Now, I am not condoning or advocating laziness. What I am saying is – let the housework (and all the other 'shoulds') take their rightful place in your life. Allow yourself to prioritise. Sometimes we do housework / chores rather than nurture ourselves in healthy ways that would leave us happier, healthier human beings. So, rather than dismissing sitting down with a good book as frivolous in the face of a messy kitchen or overgrown lawn, see it for what it is, *you nurturing you*, by taking time out for what you would truly *like* to do at that moment in time. Half and hour, or and hour later, or tomorrow, the kitchen / lawn can be dealt with. In these small ways, you can daily nurture yourself appropriately, and feed yourself emotionally by doing what you love to do, while still getting the daily chores done.

Be it knitting, or painting, dancing, writing, or watching a favourite DVD, phoning a good friend or planning a holiday, it matters not, the message is clear – **do what you love** – for it is another precious (albeit overlooked or condemned) doorway out of eating when full.

We feed ourselves emotionally when we spend time doing what we love.

We feed ourselves <u>appropriately</u> when we spend time doing what we love.

We feed ourselves <u>in</u>appropriately by eating when full.

We feed ourselves appropriately when we stop when full.

Spending time doing what we love, is a more satisfying, nurturing and appropriate way of feeding ourselves when we are not physically hungry, than eating when full,

for spending time doing what we love, truly fills the space,

that no amount, of food when full, can fill.

Physical hunger – a closer look

Feeling hungry – wanting to eat when actually physically hungry – the stomach is physically empty, either completely empty or partially empty. This hunger is a natural, healthy desire to feed and nourish the body appropriately. Eating in response to this hunger keeps us alive. If we are carrying excess weight, eating only in response to physical hunger, allows us to get slim and stay slim. If we are already slim, eating only in response to physical hunger, allows us to stay slim.

Emotional hunger – a closer look

Emotional hunger is the craving to eat even though you are already physically full, and the stomach is in the process of digesting that food. Often described as *mouth hunger* for the sensation of emotional hunger is experienced in the mouth rather than the stomach. It can be the idea that – *I've just got to put something in my mouth.* Or, *Well, it just tastes so good I must keep on eating it even though I am full.* It is a compulsion to eat, and there is a distinct difference between this *craving or compulsion to eat* when physically full and the *healthy desire to eat* as a result of genuine physical hunger. The difference between these two 'hunger' states is what you will be familiarising yourself with, in the first few weeks and months of altering and changing your eating habits.

Eating when physically full, or eating in response to emotional hunger is what makes us fat!

I cannot emphasise this enough - Asking yourself – What feeling is this? And then – Given the fact I feel this way what would I like to do now? – is the appropriate way to deal with emotional hunger.

As previously mentioned, this emotional hunger or craving food when already physically full, is the conscious or subconscious urge to suppress uncomfortable feelings. Eating when physically full is an inappropriate yet often automatic response to emotional hunger, and it is the trap that makes us fat.

The persistent and consistent practice of the aforementioned **Am I hungry?** assignment, helps develop an awareness that ultimately leads to being easily able to distinguish between physical and emotional hunger, to such a degree, that the difference will be as clear to you, as the difference between night and day, an essential part of what gets, and keeps, us slim.

I now let *being physically hungry* be my guide as to *when I eat.*

I now let *what I fancy eating* be my guide as to *what I eat.*

I now let *being physically full* be my guide as to *when to stop eating.*

Favourite foods and food we fancy

I also encourage you to keep your favourite foods in the kitchen. Eating whatever you want, when you want, as long as you are physically hungry, is made easier by having an ample larder, and reassuring yourself that the only **fattening food is food when full**.

It is important to no longer deny ourselves our favourite foods, and to allow ourselves to eat those foods that have been labelled as 'fattening' if that is what we fancy eating when we are genuinely physically hungry. Let me reassure you, that I've been naturally slim for over twenty years now, and I eat those foods that have been labelled *fattening foods* – there is not a food on this planet that I deny myself, for I know, if I did, soon I'd be bingeing on it. So permission is the key here. If I fancy it, and I'm genuinely physically hungry, then I eat it until I don't want any more of that particular food or I'm full, but without exception, I stop when full. That is how I got slim, and why I've been slim for over twenty years – I stop when I'm full.

So, have courage, and as much as you can, stock up on that chocolate ice cream, your favourite snacks, and whatever foods you've been busily denying yourself in the name of weight loss. Have the fruit and veg in aswell, along with tins, packets and frozen. If you feel some trepidation, you are not alone, for most people fear this *stocking up on the goodies* assignment, simply because they fear that they would not be able to resist eating all this food at once, and as a result, gain even more weight. And this is a valid fear, but we are *facing that fear* by having an abundance of those foods around us, and available to us. We are learning to trust ourselves around that previously forbidden food, and trust is ultimately going to replace fear.

We are truly testing our ability to *only eat when physically hungry and stop when physically full* by having all that tempting food around. The heat is on, if you like, when the previously forbidden food is suddenly available like never before. Many women resist this idea but let's face the issue squarely – When has, not having yummy food in the house stopped us from going on a binge? When we want to binge, we will go out and buy all that forbidden food, as soon as we have the opportunity to do so.

So, have some of your favourite foods in the house, and reassure yourself that you *can* eat it *if you are already physically hungry and that is what you fancy eating at that moment in time,* but stopping when full is your all-important aim.

And please remember: Food does not have the power to trigger a binge, an unresolved emotional issue and the compulsion to *stuff it down,* does. Whether or not the food is readily available, is a side issue in what it is going to take, to way-lay a binge. And to further reassure you, here are some wise words on the subject, from Susie Orbach, author of 'Fat is a Feminist Issue' and 'Susie Orbach On Eating.'

'If certain foods worry you, if sweets, bread or bananas scare you, try having enough or that particular food around so that you can never eat it all.

If you think you could binge on:

3 chocolate bars

a packet of biscuits

a pot of chocolate moose

keep 8 or 10 times as many of them in the house.

This may seem a strange thing to try but this is how to change the mystique associated with these foods. If you have plenty of them around, more than you could possibly eat in one go, you will start to see them as just foods you enjoy, foods that are staples to have when you are hungry for them.'

If, when you are physically hungry, you find yourself only wanting to eat chocolate for a greater part of the time (as I did) – allow yourself to eat it, and simply keep on practicing stopping when full, before long, you'll be saying to yourself – *I don't actually want to live off this stuff!*

It is an extremely important turning point when we realise the following:

1. We have the power to *stop when full* even with the yummy food around.

2. That we actually do <u>not</u> want to live off sugar, chocolate, ice cream, or carbohydrate for the rest of our days.

Paradoxically, these realisations only come *after we give up denying ourselves* the very foods we've been busily avoiding. Moderation kicks in with real power, automatically here, from your own joyous, wise, knowing, inner directive, that you are happy to follow, as opposed to self-denial, a self-imposed, forced directive that you really do not want to follow.

It's like the well-known stories of people who have worked in sweet shops or chocolate factories, and their boss says – 'Go ahead, eat as much as you like!' Their first reaction is – 'Great I can eat as much chocolate as I like!' However within a fortnight, they are quite happy to refuse that bar of chocolate in favour of healthier food. They know that they can eat as much chocolate as they want, and they see that there is so much of it that they couldn't possibly eat it all in one go. They have had a direct experience of how it *feels* to overindulge on sugar and chocolate, and it is not that pleasant. They know from direct experience that you can enjoy a bar of chocolate, but to eat more and more of it in one go, leaves you feeling sickly, sluggish and can give you pimples. So they learn through direct experience that they don't want it half as much as they thought they would. Give yourself this valuable experience, either by getting a job in a sweet shop, or by stocking up on your favourite foods. It may be hard to believe, but it bears repeating - having your favourite food in the house, doesn't cause a binge half as much as old, ineffective habits, unresolved emotional issues, and forced denial of our favourite foods when genuinely physically hungry. Let's also remind ourselves that controlling our food intake, through forced denial of our favourite foods when genuinely physically hungry for them, and ignoring our feelings, does nothing to help us heal our food addiction. It is those concepts that are part of what cause, and perpetuate food addiction.

We are affirming that we deserve to have the food we like, available to us when we are physically hungry for them. We are displaying a trust in ourselves to nourish our bodies appropriately, and only eat when physically hungry. We are also, quite literally, trusting ourselves to be around the object of our addiction without indulging in it. Whereas, if we continue to keep our cupboards empty except for a packet of diet crackers and a low-cal milk shake, when the urge to binge strikes, we will notice how we zoom down to the local 24 hour shop to buy-a-binge. So, let's really acknowledge, that an empty kitchen has never really helped us cease eating when physically full, and the truth of the matter is, that if we do manage to eat only when physically hungry and stop when physically full, even though all that tempting food is in the house, then we are definitely no longer compulsive eaters, or food junkies.

Restricting or forbidding our favourite foods – recap

1. Restricting and forbidding ourselves our favourite foods, when we are actually, genuinely, physically hungry, does not help us lose weight, in fact it creates the climate in which the tendency to binge on them is increased, for the minute we say – 'I can't have that!' We want it all the more.

2. Restricting and forbidding ourselves our favourite foods when we are actually physically hungry for them, gives those foods a magical meaning, a forbidden essence, which in turn makes them

all the more desirable, and the tendency to binge on them is increased. We tend to become obsessed with the foods we want but actively deny ourselves when physically hungry.

3.   Forced denial of calorie-laden foods when we are genuinely physically hungry, usually results in overindulgence on them, when full, at a later date.

Now, I am not condoning a lack of self-discipline here in saying let yourself have an abundance of your favourite foods in the house. I am laying down a guideline, which, when followed, leads to natural and permanent slimness. We are finding a balance between over-indulgence and strict denial. If we are doing any denying here it is this – denying ourselves food when full. And, if fact, the use of the word 'deny' in this context, is slightly inaccurate. When we are physically full and still crave to eat more, it is ineffective to simply forcibly deny ourselves *food when full* at that moment, it is shaky ground, an unstable foundation to build your slimness on. Forced abstention from what is, in reality, the object of your addiction (food when full) usually backfires, for it is like forcing yourself to give up your means of coping with your un-addressed, emotional issues and uncomfortable feelings. Following the principles of permission, choice and understanding, is the kinder, more effective way, creating a solid foundation on which to be slim. Let us explore these concepts:

Permission – permission to eat when full if you really want to, makes it easier to choose not to.

Choice – the choice to eat what foods you want to eat when genuinely physically hungry, and the choice to <u>not</u> eat when full is increased by resolving emotional issues.

Understanding – understanding that eating when full is a coping mechanism, and sometimes we are going to use that old coping mechanism until the new coping mechanism is firmly in place (as provided by the **Am I hungry?** assignment).

When you think of it, many, many people in this world do <u>not</u> have the compulsion to eat when full. I *used to* have the compulsion to eat when full, but not any more, and that is <u>directly because</u>, I have been aware of, felt, and dealt with, the underlying emotional stuff that was causing me to *want* to eat when full. In other words, being aware of, feeling, and dealing with my underlying emotional stuff, aswell as giving myself permission to eat whatever I fancied when physically hungry, actually caused me to no longer crave the object of my addiction – food when full. No longer craving food when full, meant I no longer ate when full, so I got slim and stayed slim. A powerful combination of ideas, providing a dynamic way forward, in short - addiction-busting, strategies.

When you no longer crave food when full you no longer bother with food when full.

- I allow myself to eat whatever I fancy when I am physically hungry.

- I understand that *food when full* puts on weight.

- I understand that *food when full* stuffs down my uncomfortable feelings / unresolved emotional stuff.

- I understand that *food when full* is an object of addiction just like drugs, alcohol, gambling, smoking etc.

- I allow myself to give up all objects of addiction now.

- I know that *feeling my feelings* is what happens when I give up *eating when full*.

- I know that asking myself – Given the fact I feel this way, what would I like to do now? – helps me resolve my feelings / emotional stuff.

- I now *resolve* rather than *stuff down* my feelings.

- I now stop when full, and as a result, get slim, and stay slim.

Assignment – List in a notebook all the foods you deny yourself:

Example:

Garlic bread

Chocolate biscuits

Now, let yourself stock up on, one, two or three of these forbidden foods as extra items this week. They must be the exact foods that you have been denying yourself, food that you maybe never allow yourself to have in the house. You know the ones, bread, chocolate muffins, tortilla chips, and as Susie Orbach says, '…buy enough of it so that you could not possibly eat it all in one sitting.' Your aim is to simply eat it when you are physically hungry and fancy it.

Often, the only time we allow ourselves the high calorie, foods we fancy, is when we are on a binge, and a part of us knows that when the binge is over – that's it, no more yummy foods – and it is back to the lettuce leaf, in the name of ever-elusive, slimness. What a riot, what a game that has never empowered us to lose weight for good. So, let's drop the restriction with confidence, and allow ourselves the food we love, that includes sweet food, savoury food, frozen food, tined food, packet food, dried food, fresh food, spicy food and bland food. And simply *trust* ourselves, to choose which ones to eat, when genuinely physically hungry, knowing that we will stop when simply full and not when absolutely stuffed. As we endeavour to do this, we soon discover that the urge to binge has very little to do with what food is or isn't in the house, and a lot to do with how we are feeling emotionally.

True Slimness Weight Loss Principle # 6 We no longer deny ourselves the foods we fancy when physically hungry.

How can I stop when full?

Okay, now that we have established that 'will-power' is a bit-player in this game of being able to stop when full, and are focusing our attention on what really empowers us to stop when simply full - the aforementioned, all-important, assignment - **Am I hungry?** I would like to expand on it a little:

Aswell as asking – Given the fact I feel this way what would I like to do now? You can also ask yourself the following questions to gain even more clarity and aid resolving:

- What situation / person / event is this about?

- What words can best describe how I am feeling right now?

- Is this feeling 'held' somewhere in my body, such as a tightness in my throat or butterflies in my stomach?

See if you can simply observe your feelings without getting too caught up in them, so to speak, or overwhelmed by them. Watch them as it were, notice how they come and go. We cannot always act on our feelings, so gaining practice at just *feeling the intensity of the feelings* is a valuable tool, and a fine art, which makes life without overeating, possible.

It is a subtle shift you are making in the way you relate to yourself, food, and feelings. There is no getting away from feelings, we are human, and we are going to have feelings as part of our day-to-day living. Just as a day has weather, a human has feelings. Some of us, for the most part deny or suppress our feelings, and some of us, for the most part acknowledge and feel our feelings. This is a huge difference that we are talking about here, and what you are discovering is - How to be people, who, for the most part, acknowledge and feel their feelings, and thus, can gain freedom from compulsive eating and other addictions. Yes, what I am teaching is a change of tactics in how to deal with uncomfortable feelings – The change from suppression (eating when full) to feeling (stopping when full).

So, as you feel your feelings and practice the **Am I hungry?** assignment daily, you might be surprised at the interesting and sometimes very simple ideas that spring to mind as a means of resolving your various emotional issues. Follow through on what seems appropriate in answer to – 'Given the fact I feel this way what would I like to do now?' – for this simple method, when put into practice, enables you to resolve your own problems, feelings and emotional stuff. And it empowers you to meet life's challenges with greater ease.

Remember, getting slim does not necessarily mean life gets any easier. When slim you could have the exact same problems as you have now, or you could have different ones, and maybe even a few that you would consider quite difficult or unmanageable. The thing is, and this is a vitally important difference – you will be *handling those challenges in different ways,* ways that you are learning and practicing now, through reading this book. Soon you will no longer be eating when full and suppressing feelings and intuition, you will be meeting your own emotional needs throughout any challenge. This is the *new habit* you are already getting into, replacing the old weight gaining habit of eating when full. The new habit allows, what once felt monumental, or was so deeply suppressed that you were not even aware of it to be easily dealt with, and resolved for good, and you move on to brighter and better things!

Cravings to eat when full are dissolved as feelings are felt and resolved.

And so, step-by-step, we are able to feel our feelings and deal with our emotional issues, rather than eat when full / binge eat because of them. As a direct result of eating when physically hungry and stopping when physically full, our bodies are able to permanently establish their own natural weight. Both the original emotional issues that caused us to overeat, and the problem of excess weight, have been dealt with, effectively. As we no longer need to eat when full because of emotional issues, the addiction, to food when full, is healed.

True Slimness Weight Loss Principle # 7 We eat when full because of unmet needs. Stopping when full, involves meeting needs.

Example: You have just eaten a hot meal you really enjoyed. You allowed yourself to eat exactly what you wanted and stopped when you were simply full. You are now sitting in front of the T.V and you are finishing off a mug of coffee and a chocolate biscuit. You realise you want to eat more biscuits. You feel the urge to get up and go into the kitchen in search of the biscuit tin. You ask yourself the question you have been repeatedly using: **Am I hungry?** The answer comes – No. You check in with your stomach, noticing how it feels – It feels full. You notice the craving to eat more biscuits even though you are full. This moment is crucial:

- This is the moment in time, that you are physically full yet still crave to eat more.

- This is the moment in time, that you are considering eating when full.

- This is the moment in time, that you are compelled to indulge in the eating that is the direct cause of excess weight – eating when full.

- This is the moment in time, that you are drawn to indulge in that which you are trying to abstain from – eating when full.

- This is the moment in time, when, if you allow yourself to wait until you are physically hungry before eating again, you will be putting your body in the position, whereby it can actually start to shed the excess weight you are carrying, for it is through *stopping when full* that the body both finds and keeps its own natural weight.

This, in no uncertain terms, is your power-point, (what I repeatedly speak about in this book, for it is your key to true and lasting slimness). It is at this exact moment in time – when you are physically full but crave to eat more, that you can ask yourself: **What feeling is this?** And: **Given the fact I feel this way, what would I like to do now?** The answer to which arms you with the alternative to eating when full. Thus providing yourself with the appropriate means of coping with your feelings and emotional issues.

Back to our example: You notice that you are feeling dissatisfied with your living arrangements, especially your flatmate with whom you have had several arguments. Now that you have realised how you are feeling emotionally (dissatisfied), and what the issue is (either put up with your flatmate or move out) – you ask yourself – **Given the fact I feel this way what would I like to do**

now? You look around and realise that you have grown somewhat tired of the flat and would not miss it too much if you left. You notice you have a strong desire to move out, and even though fear has always stopped you before, you resolve to look for a new flat. You decide you will buy the papers tomorrow to see what flats are available. In this way you have resolved your emotional issue, the one that was at the root of that urge to eat biscuits when full.

As you can see, this is a much more freeing way to deal with what life presents us with. Be it a grumpy flat mate or some other issue, we simply know, that whatever life gives us, can be dealt with in ways other than eating when we are, in truth, physically full. So life becomes a little different because of this shift in our ways of relating to ourselves, our feelings, and our world. It is a more empowering standpoint. You have more choice, and you are making the healthier choice – the choice to live rather than suppress.

We are, in effect, learning which feelings to act upon, and which feelings to sit with and allow to pass, as well as different ways of acting on any given feeling.

When, for example you feel anger, you may *feel* like slapping your husband but you do not act on it. *That,* is a feeling that would be healthier (and less abusive to your husband) to act on in a different way, such as going out immediately for a brisk walk, or going to the nearest toilet to do a silent scream, both good ways to deal with anger – safe, effective, non-abusive ways. Whereas, if you find yourself feeling overwhelming love for your husband, then, that is a good feeling to act on in the obvious way!

Eating when hungry and stopping when full – written assignment:

In a notebook write down the answers to the following question – In general, what would you say are the main feelings and emotional issues that cause you to binge / eat when full? (List at least three).

Example: *Stress and boredom cause me to eat when full, also I fear my husband might be having an affair. When he rings to say he is working late, I always binge eat once the kids are in bed.*

Okay, look at your list and really acknowledge that it is hard for you to stop eating when full when you are experiencing these feelings and faced with that particular issue. Really take time to acknowledge, that eating when physically full has been your way of coping with this emotional stuff, and that resolving these issues is going to be a big part of your life as you get smaller.

Feeling and resolving gets bigger as I get smaller

Over a period of a week, carry a small notebook around with you, notice and write a few lines when these or other issues arise:

Example # 1: *Tuesday – I felt so stressed when I was taking the kids to the park, I simply did not have enough sleep the night before, and my son started to cry, so I took them to the shop to buy them ice-cream and, even though I was full (I had just had a large dinner and desert) I bought and ate, three chocolate bars and a packet of crisps, I also kept on eating when I got home.*

Example # 2: *Wednesday - My husband phoned to say he'd be late home from work. I immediately felt suspicious and angry. I went up to the bedroom and got down on my knees and beat the mattress with my fists. I kept on thinking 'It's not fair, it's not fair,' and then a strange thing came to mind, I remembered when I was little and my mother not letting me out to play with the neighbourhood kids, and feeling the same thing – trapped! I then asked myself – 'Given the fact I feel this way, what would I like to do now?' And I washed my face and took the kids down to the local library, which is open until 8pm. I noticed I felt very free striding down the road pushing the double buggy, the children happy, and me aware of the cool, late summer evening air on my face. We had a lovely time at the library, I even bumped into one of the Mum's who goes to the same Mother and Toddler group as we do. We enjoyed a chat, and our children played, I borrowed a copy of 'Loving What Is,' by Byron Katie and the picture books my children choose, and we spent a lovely evening in when we got home, reading until the children fell asleep. I then did some of the written work from Byron Katie's book and found it helped me feel clearer about the situation – I didn't feel great, but I did not binge.* (Please do keep your notebook private and in a safe place, so only you can see your notes about your thoughts and feelings.)

Then, when you have a quiet moment, consider how you handled those emotional issues, feelings and events. In the first example, you might simply acknowledge that your old means of coping (eating when full) was what you used *that* day, to help you deal with how you were feeling - forgive yourself, know that it is okay to make mistakes. Hindsight is a wonderful thing, and a healing thing too, when, any time we've eaten when full because of our emotional stuff, we ask ourselves, while looking back on the event - What other way could I have reacted to those emotions and issues as they arose? Write down your answers, and take a moment to visualise yourself handling the matter in a much more effective way, a way that did not involve you eating when physically full. This paves the way for future success.

If you have an experience like in example number two, then congratulate yourself for resisting the urge to binge and finding the healthy alternative (beating the mattress, and then a walk to the library) through asking – Given the fact I feel this way what would I like to do now?

By doing this simple assignment, you are reinforcing in your mind, the idea that there are *other ways,* of confronting, the day-to-day challenges of life. You are reinforcing the idea that you *can* give up eating when full as a habitual way of being, acting, and reacting. You are giving yourself a choice, opening a door for yourself. That door may not be that easy to open, and the path beyond it, may not always be that smooth, and it certainly isn't a familiar path, it is, as yet, unknown, but it is the pathway of no binges, and true and lasting slimness. A new and exciting route to take!

What gets you slim, keeps you slim – stopping when full!

In my own experience, healing the habit of binge eating, being able to stop when full, I found out that on this unknown path, small steps were the order of the day until the inevitable, quantum leap would take place in interesting and often surprising ways. But the first step was to get into the habit of asking (this bears repeating) **Am I physically hungry?** The next step was, one by one, handling the nuances of my life in slightly different ways, while allowing the strengthening of my recognition, or awareness of my own *degrees of hunger,* and *degrees of fullness,* as I continued to listen to the sensations of my stomach.

In the subsequent years of working with compulsive eaters, it also became evident to me that it is sometimes useful to describe the individual degrees of physical hunger and fullness:

Degree 1 of hunger – The peckish feeling – this arises when the stomach is about half, or three quarters full. There is room to comfortably eat a little bit more before feeling completely full. It can be described as – *I fancy a hot drink and a slice of toast and marmalade* – and you would feel completely full afterwards. A small amount of food satisfies that peckish sensation. It could be a biscuit and a coffee half an hour after a meal, or a banana shortly after breakfast, or half a portion of chips that you share with a friend or your child. Your inner directive will, as always, guide you.

Degree 2 of hunger – A bit more hungry than simply feeling peckish – this usually happens when the stomach is about half empty. You could comfortably go without eating for another hour or so, until more serious hunger sensations appear. You could eat a small amount comfortably before feeling physically full. As with the peckish sensation, eating or not eating, is equally comfortable at this degree of hunger.

Degree 3 of hunger – This can be described as – *I'm starving!* This type of hunger occurs when the stomach really is empty, and needs more food in the form of a substantial meal, right now. It is this ravenous sensation that occurs when the stomach is physically empty and it's been several hours (usually four or more) since you last ate anything. If you are extremely hungry, you may experience shaking, a drop in blood sugar, have a headache, feel faint or lightheaded. When you are *this* hungry and still refuse to eat, your metabolism could start to slow down. It is a kickback to primitive times. A survival mechanism built into the body to help deal with food shortages or famine.

You see, in caveman times, the only reason primitive man or woman would not eat when physically hungry, was, if they could not find food, or were unsuccessful on the hunt. Physical hunger, was the hunger they automatically acted on by eating until they were full, they wouldn't dream of not eating when physically hungry. It shows how dysfunctional our eating patterns are, when we think it is a good idea to go against this inner wisdom.

Now, Mother Nature, in her wisdom did not want humans who could not find food to be in danger of immediate starvation, that is why she set in place, the automatic, *slowing down of metabolism* under the conditions of *non-eating when hungry*. That way, if food was scarce, the human race would still survive until food was more plentiful again. With a slow metabolism you are talking double calories when you eat again, and so, if we starve and binge (an eating habit I had throughout my teenage years) we are really setting ourselves up for weight gain, both through the eating when full, and the slowed metabolism from the period of not eating when hungry.

Mother Nature probably never imagined that we humans could get things so mixed up, as to choose to actively ignore a healthy impulse to eat when genuinely, physically hungry. The impulse that She put there to ensure things run smoothly weight wise.

So please remind yourself often, that going long periods of time (like most of the day) without eating, does little or nothing to help and overweight person lose weight, it only serves to slow the metabolism down. It is amazing to think that so many of us have gone hours and hours, maybe even a good part of the day without eating, thinking that in so doing, we were losing weight, when all we were doing was magically doubling the calorific value of the food we eventually did eat, and thus we inadvertently *increased* our chances of gaining weight – that's what happens when we ignore our hunger sensations.

We can hopefully now see, the beautiful balance, and intricacy that is already in place within our very own hunger and fullness sensations that are simply there, to guide us, in the most healthy way as to when to eat, and when to stop eating, and in abiding by them, lose the excess weight. So let's stop starving ourselves thinking it will help us lose weight, and instead, abide by the natural balance of – I'm hungry, I eat. I'm full, I stop eating.

True Slimness Weight loss Principle # 8 Not eating when genuinely physically hungry messes about with your metabolism. Eating when hungry and stopping when full is all about being kind to your body.

- No more the extreme of not eating when physically hungry
- No more the extreme of eating when full.
- Now the natural balance of I am hungry, I eat. I am full, I stop eating.
- Feeling discomfort when we overeat, is the body's way of telling us, *eating when full is a bad idea.*
- Eating when the body tells us to eat and in stopping when the body tells us to stop is being kind to the body.

Degree 1 of fullness – This can be described as *just taking the edge off my hunger*. After eating, we no longer really feel hungry, but probably will feel hungry again in an hour or two. This degree of fullness involves eating only a light snack, or as little as half a pack of crisps. In other words, a few mouthfuls of food, or slightly more, you will find, will give you this degree of fullness.

We can be *on the move* when we eat like this. In a busy day, this type of eating is great, it does not require any necessary 'sit down and rest' after eating, that a large meal can require. Another attribute of stopping at this degree of fullness, is that you could comfortably *eat more without feeling stuffed*, and also, it is not uncomfortable to wait another hour or two before eating again, because you already, feel satisfied having stopped at that point. *Eating little and often* can be the pattern that emerges when we continually stop at this degree of fullness, and it is a fine pattern of eating, perfectly healthy, and slim friendly.

Degree 2 of fullness – Eating more that just enough to cover your hunger pangs, you begin to *fill up with food*, but not to the extent that you are in any way stuffed. You are simply *comfortably full*. You could get up and enjoy a stroll, or a countryside walk after this degree of fullness. Jogging would be out of the question, and only another few mouthfuls of food, would take you to the, *not another bite,* sensation.

Degree 3 of fullness – This is the, *not another bite,* fullness. You are physically full, and if you have *another* few mouthfuls or more, you may feel stuffed or bloated. This is the type of fullness that, whilst still comfortable, you would like to sit down and rest after eating. You would probably gain some weight at this degree of fullness.

Degree 4 of fullness – This is the fullness sensation we get when we overeat, ignoring and overriding all the previous fullness sensations. Tummy ache, feeling bloated, stuffed or nauseous are some of the signals coming from the stomach. We feel this type of fullness after a binge. The stomach is physically expanded beyond its natural capabilities - it is, quite literally, self-abuse. It is a strain on the internal organs to physically cope with that much food. We have ignored all of the previous fullness sensations telling us to stop eating. Consciously or subconsciously, this overeating has been triggered by an unresolved emotional issue and having no other way of dealing with it, we felt out of control and were absolutely unable to stop eating. This food will be turned into fat, but can be absorbed when we master the art of stopping eating at the 1st and 2nd degree of fullness.

Another issue that arises as we practice the fine art of eating when hungry and stopping when full, is that sometimes, we are not sure exactly, what it is, that our stomach is trying to tell us. Is that the sensation of being genuinely, physically hungry, or is it emotional hunger i.e. the craving to eat when full? What to do in a case like this? – Experiment!

Hungry but not sure – Option 1 – Eat

Eat – When you think you feel *physical hunger but are not sure* – eat, and simply notice how your stomach feels as you are eating. If you are stuffed after a few mouthfuls then that *hunger sensation* may have really been emotional hunger, you were actually physically full, and <u>not</u> in need of food, but in need of comfort, or some form of emotional release or resolving.

Hungry but not sure – Option 2 - Don't Eat – When you think you feel *physical hunger* but are not sure – don't eat, and simply notice how the stomach feels about this <u>absence</u> of food and eating. If you are ravenous within half an hour, then you really were physically hungry and it would have been fine to eat what you fancied until physically full at that moment in time, when you initially had that hunger pang. So, with hindsight, you are gaining familiarity with these subtle degrees of hunger and fullness. Fine tuning your awareness and recognition of them, until you will automatically know, exactly when you are physically hungry, and exactly when you are full.

☯

Some Weighty Myths

Many people say to me – 'But I don't eat chocolate, I don't have a sweet tooth, why do I still have a weight problem?'

I tell them – 'You are presuming that chocolate alone, or sweet things alone are the cause of excess weight. The *type* of food you eat does not greatly influence your weight. The ultimate determining factor in weight gain, is not *what* you ate, but being *physically full* when you ate it.'

To further clarify the point:

Chocolate eaten when physically hungry will <u>not</u> put weight on.

Cream cakes eaten when physically hungry will <u>not</u> put weight on.

Chips eaten when physically hungry will <u>not</u> put weight on.

However:

Chocolate eaten when *physically full* <u>will</u> put weight on.

Cream cakes eaten when *physically full* <u>will</u> put weight on.

Chips eaten when *physically full* <u>will</u> put weight on.

Weighty Myth: Avoid snacking between meals.

Holistic Truth: Snacking between meals when *physically full* causes weight gain and prevents weight loss.

Holistic truth: Snacking between meals when *physically hungry* does not cause weight gain and allows weight loss.

Weighty Myth: Grazing causes excess weight.

Holistic Truth: Grazing when *physically full* causes weight gain and prevents weight loss.

Holistic Truth: Grazing when *physically hungry* does not cause weight gain and allows weight loss.

Feeling full is the body's way of saying – 'No more calories for now, no more fuel for now, I've got some excess fat to burn here!'

As you can see, the golden rule is physical hunger! Being physically hungry is the only reason to eat. So don't worry about grazing or snacking, for they cannot cause excess weight in and of themselves, as always, the deciding factor in the weight loss stakes, is being physically hungry before eating.

The main point, is to simply focus on paying attention to the hunger and fullness sensations when snacking or grazing, and eliminate any grazing or snacking when full. Know there is an emotional issue underneath that urge to graze or snack when you are already full of food, and it is in the resolving of it, that your freedom from *food when full* lies.

True Slimness Weight Loss Principle # 9 Grazing all-day and snacking between meals when *physically hungry* does not cause weight gain – snacking and grazing when full does.

Eating when hungry and stopping when full – Assignment

With a pen and paper and an undisturbed 20 mins or so, think back in time, and name and describe periods in your life, or individual events that caused you to gain weight. Emotions and memories will come up as you write and this is okay, uncomfortable but okay, let yourself feel the feelings and ask yourself – How best can I support and nurture myself as I allow myself to no longer suppress these old hurts? Take action on the ideas and jot down what happens.

Example: *When I was 24 I split up with my live-in boyfriend and was feeling so distressed I gained 10 kilos.* How can I support and nurture myself through these feelings of loss and grief that I feel now as I write about this? *I actually let myself have a good cry and did not tell myself it was silly to cry over something that happened so long ago. I felt relieved, and then decided to watch my favourite romantic comedy DVD, curled up on the sofa with the cat at my feet, I then snoozed until morning. The next day I was surprised how well I had slept, and felt I had really acknowledged and released the hurt I previously felt. I could think about it without feeling tearful.*

Example: *When I was 15, my mother came back from visiting her sister and had bought my brother and Dad a big bar of chocolate each as presents and didn't buy me one, but announced loudly that I don't want chocolate anymore because I'm always dieting! I had been looking forward to that bar of chocolate all day, she used to always buy me one, and I felt I could have eaten it in moderation. I felt so unloved and insecure I binged on apple pie. I wanted to say - I am angry at your attitude towards me Mum. I want you to love and appreciate me, not continually try to control and manipulate me. Even though I am a teenager I still need you. I was also hurt that my brother and dad did not offer to share their chocolate with me. I concluded that what I want isn't important.*

How I supported myself as I felt those old feelings again: *I felt like a walk in the fresh air, so I put the lead on the dog and took her for a walk by the river, in fact I jogged some of the way even though I wasn't wearing jogging gear, just jeans and a tee shirt! It didn't matter I felt like running and I did! And as I ran, I embraced the feeling of the anger being run off, and the cobwebs being blown away in the chillness of the breeze. I also noticed how much my beloved dog loves me unconditionally, and shed a few tears. I also did an inner-child visualisation I found on Dr Doris Cohen's web site (www.drdoriscohen.com) when I got home. That really helped me heal that wounded part of me.*

It is important to *now feel* the sorrow and pain of those past incidents as you remember them, or if they spontaneously come up during your day (as they will, when you continually stop when full). Acknowledge that, at that time, you really did not have any other way of dealing with how you were feeling emotionally, but now you do. Have compassion on who you were then, and promise yourself you will never be left with an unsatisfactory means of coping with life's difficulties. Promise yourself that you will always have a friend to ring, a park to walk in, a shoulder to cry on, or a DVD to watch. Reassure yourself that you *can* handle, without binge-eating, anything that life gives you as a challenge or uncomfortable feeling. I cannot promise you a life without heartache, but I am sharing with you, how a to have a life without food binges and excess weight because of heartache.

Communicating what we want

Sometimes our fat is declaring to the world and important message on our behalf, such as – 'Go away.' Or 'Something's wrong.' Or 'I need to protect myself.'

When we are overweight we may feel we have no way of saying what we want to say – our fat says it for us. In order to give up the fat for good, we must learn how to realise what our fat is saying for us, and then, how to say that for ourselves. This takes courage, willingness and the intention to articulate our needs. And we can do this by simply closing our eyes and doing some daydreaming....

Simply, take a few undisturbed minutes, sit in a comfortable chair, relax and imagine yourself in your usual day to day routine, and all the while, have in mind, this question – 'What is my excess weight saying to these people?'

You may have to do this a few times over the period of a week to get any clear ideas about what your excess weight is trying to communicate for you, or you might immediately get insights. That does not matter; simply allow it to unfold in its own time. And once you have your insights then ask yourself – 'How can I communicate this verbally and / or through my actions?' – And daydream about doing that. You are communicating the message to your mind – Hey, look you can deal with this situation in this new way.

Our excess weight might be saying to our spouse – 'Be there for me.' Or to an emotionally distant mother – 'I forgive you.' It could be saying to your best friend - 'Look, I'm not a threat to your marriage.' There are many, many unspoken messages contained in the fat cells of your body, now is the time to discover them, while letting go of the excess weight, which did not have the power to adequately communicate them anyway, at least not in a way that would allow you to be slim.

Example: *My fat is screaming to my husband – Help me around the house more!*

How can I communicate this? *I can ask my husband to always do the washing up every Tuesday night so I can get an early night. I have never been specific in my requests before, always just* *complaining. If he still refuses, or agrees and then does not do it, I will simply employ a cleaner two mornings a week, my friend has one that she says is really good.*

So there we are, finding the hidden messages our fat was trying to say for us, and taking that step into the unknown territory of *voicing our own requests to get our needs met.* This does not mean others will always comply, or that we should try to control or manipulate the folk in our life. These messages are about needs, preferences and wishes, and can indeed be communicated, and deemed important enough for us to act on in such a way as to get our needs met, our preferences taken into consideration, and our wishes fulfilled in a way that benefits everyone, and suppress no feelings, and oppresses no one.

In a further effort to acknowledge and meet our own emotional needs in life, we need to ask ourselves:

What do I need to gain in my life instead of excess weight?

What do I need to lose in my life as well as excess weight?

What sweetness would I love more of, in my life, instead of sweet foods when full?

How do I deal with life's bitter experiences?

How do I cope when things go sour? Are there any new and better ways I could employ?

What is the best case scenario in this situation concerning ....?

I often feel it is key, that it is through the throat, the centre of communication, that food is pushed into an already full stomach, in the dysfunctional effort to get our needs met. The throat is the place from which we utter our words, phrases and everyday conversations. Eating when full is like stuffing down those very words that might help us express and resolve what is bothering us. When we give up this eating when physically full, it is like we free up the throat, the words and level of communication alters and changes to one where we are more able to voice our opinions. We are able to say those words we did not say before. It could be saying, *I love you,* to a cherished mate, or, *I will not tolerate you speaking to me that way,* to a family member or spouse. Something is liberated within us through the cessation of that activity that stuffed our words and feelings down.

We are now learning how to feel our feelings without cringing, or shame but with the sure knowledge that our feelings are linked to our episodes of binge eating, and therefore, to sort our eating out, we have got to sort our feelings out, and in sorting our feelings out, we sort our lives out, and that involves, allowing certain words out.

No more not enough of this and too much of that, we are seeking, finding, and establishing true balance in our lives by asking for what we want and know to be right and true for us personally on a daily basis, food wise, emotionally, and practically, in each area of our life. And, as we keep doing what it takes to healthily fulfil our own individual needs, we actually experience getting our needs met, and feel the satisfaction of a job well done on our own behalf.

I realise that many, many women fear that this is being selfish, so I ask you, what happens when we do the opposite, and <u>not</u> follow what we feel is right and true for ourselves? Well, we usually end up doing what someone else wants us to do. Our spouse, a family member, or a slightly controlling parent, like a father that wants his son to be a doctor, when the son has a great love of painting, and would rather go to Art College. Or a wife that wants to take an evening class, and her husband flatly refuses to be home on time to mind the kids for those two hours. Do you really think this sort of thing can really help anyone, or bring happiness, or even be deemed of as a good idea? Of course not. So finding a way to live life on our own terms is part and parcel of recovering from compulsive eating and being overweight. Not always easy, but not inevitably hard either, there simply *is* a way, you just have to find, and live, your own, unique, individual way. Paul McKenna has described one of the attributes of being a 'rich thinker' as being able *to - live life on your own terms.* I love this! And this we can do no matter how much money is in our bank account, for, in truth, all it depends on is *creativity* and a *willingness to find a way.*

The difference between *what you know to be right and true for you,* and what another *thinks to be right and true for you,* is what has the power to make your life, quite literally, either a joy or a misery. When you know the difference, and make a choice that is in alignment with your own heart-felt desires, this leads to your own personal happiness, although you could have a few miffed relatives along the way, they will soon come round, because people have a tendency to admire (however begrudgingly) the person who stands up for herself. If this does not happen, you may find yourself simply growing naturally apart as life continues to take you both on different paths, making room in your life for happier, healthier more supportive folk to be around. This is the way to freedom, success and true and lasting slimness, for our heart-felt desires *are* our guidance system into our own authentic life, and I for one, do not think any of us have the right to snuff that out. An authentic life, is a candle well worth watching over, and tending to.

We have free will, let us choose our own authentic life through following that which we love, interests, pursuits, studies and work, for the truth is, that nothing of real value is ever lost during the move to a more authentic way of being, a way of being in line with your heart-felt desires. Happiness is your birthright, and this is how you claim it, follow what you love, and see the story unfold. This is really where stopping when full, being more aware of our feelings, acting healthily on our feelings, communicating our needs, can and does take us. We reveal the life of our deepest longings to be a reality that is very much within our grasp. So the message is clear – Follow your own Star – not the one someone else is pointing to, saying - *follow this one instead.*

This is an individual journey, and each one of us has different needs, obligations and challenges. You may be a busy single woman with work commitments, or you may be married with little ones totally dependant on you to be that strong, reliable, fully functional provider of their needs too. You have got to come from a *full* place to do that, and to come from a full place you have got to make sure your needs are met, that includes emotional, spiritual, physical and practical. In short, you need to support you, and having, or developing, a lovely, like-minded circle of friends is so possible and worthwhile in the establishing of a life that works really well. This demands that you be *in touch with* your feelings, values, desires and needs, as well as *developing and expanding your ability* to happily deal with your feelings, desires, values and needs without getting overwhelmed. This is no small task, but it starts with being aware, and being able to communicate. Stuffing your feelings down through compulsive eating is like a brick wall between you and that loving, supported, and fulfilled life. Let this book be your sledgehammer to that brick wall, so you can move forward into the freedom of emotional resolving and its positive spin off - slimness.

To waist, for not to waste

No, I have not spelt it wrong, and forgive me Shakespeare for this very accurate pun on several concepts that we seem to have gotten all mixed up within society in general as regards food and wastage. Let us consider it this way: When physically full, instead of putting leftover food in the bin (what some would call wasting it) we have been putting it *on our waists* as excess fat, by putting it into our already full, stomachs.

Food put into our already full stomachs will get turned directly into fat cells, deposited on the body.

To put food on our waist as fat, by eating food when full in order not to waste it – is the greatest waste of all.

So, if you have been guilty of this, I am asking you now, to seriously revaluate what wastage means to you. The next time you are full, and face half a plateful of food still to be eaten, that is the time to ask yourself – Which is the greater waste, to abuse myself by shovelling that half a plateful of food into my already full stomach, or to stop when full, wrap it in cling film and put it in the fridge, or even bin it? Please remember - You are not a human dustbin!

Still we find it hard to escape the messages that *food when full to avoid wastage is a good thing.* Often this is fuelled by feelings of guilt over wastage, which were originally given to us repeatedly, by our parents, so as to encourage us to eat, even though, we may have been, rather full. However, we can deal with and overcome this conditioning, so we no longer feel compelled to eat when physically full due to guilt over wasting food. Write out on a post-it note the following weight loss principle, and stick it on your kitchen bin if necessary, to help you acknowledge the truth about wastage.

True Slimness Weight Loss Principle # 10 It is okay to bin it if I am full! I am not a human dustbin!

Western wastage and world hunger are serious issues that emerge repeatedly in my workshops and one to one sessions. So, let us look at the truth of the matter and get some clarity – Being obese does not stop world hunger! How many of us were encouraged to eat that extra spoonful of food, far beyond our natural fullness sensation, whilst being reminded of some starving child somewhere? Millions of us!

There is wastage of food in the world, but us stuffing in *food when full* is not going to solve this serious problem. If it is in your stomach when your stomach is stuffed, it does not mean waste hasn't happened. The more you empower yourself to stop when full, even if that involves binning some food, then the better equipped you are to deal with, not only your own individual feelings and issues, but also the global feelings and issues. There is a longstanding global feeling of *something needs to be done about the starving in our world,* and rightly so. I feel the way forward starts in both individually and collectively, an inner and outer resolving occurring, and that can happen when we relate to ourselves, our planet, and our fellow human beings, in a more nurturing way.

The flip side of the - 'There are millions starving in the world' coin, is - 'There are millions obese in the world.' And both these issues can be addressed. Let us look a little more at the origins of obesity, the learning to eat when full: We may have been the children whose mother was not really listening when her child said – 'No thanks Mum, I am full.' By thus ignoring our exclamations of fullness, and actively overriding our bodies natural fullness sensation, our well-meaning mothers, set the blueprint for future overriding of fullness sensations, to be done, by none other than ourselves. In other words we learned a habit – the habit of eating when full.

- To eat when full became normal.

- For eating when full we may have got praised.

- Unfortunately, eating when full, made us overweight.

So if you repeatedly demand 'empty plates' from your children when they are physically full, you are actively encouraging within them a lack of trust in their own ability, to recognise and act appropriately, on their own sensations, of physical fullness. If you find yourself doing this, it is probably just a repetition of your own upbringing. So do not be too hard on yourself, recognise your actions, forgive yourself and resolve to change. If you do not, you could be contributing to your own child's eating disorder.

True Slimness Weight Loss Principle # 11 Food has a symbolic meaning for us.

The symbolic meaning of food

A coffee can conjure up the idea of a dynamic businesswoman about to close an all-important deal, or a dinner party, with all its sophistication, glamour, companionship, and promise of romance in exotic locations. A chocolate bar can be a break, a treat and an energiser in a busy day. Cake can be a luxury, or a homely indulgence. We need to notice if we are eating when physically full because of an unmet need. Notice times that you might be relying on that product to supply the solution. This is a very ineffective and dysfunctional way to meet a very real need. When you find yourself regularly drawn to a particular food, especially the ones mentioned above, do ask yourself – What does this food symbolise for me? And – How can I bring, what it symbolises, into my life? And take some action in accordance with meeting that need. This will provide you with the answer to that need, and less of a reason to eat when full.

Other reasons why we eat when full

This may stem from childhood. How many parents repeatedly gave a chocolate bar to a crying child when a hug and a few soothing words would have been more appropriate? The result – As adults, when there is no hug available, when we are sad or depressed, we may still turn to the chocolate bar, or five! Also:

- Eating because it is teatime or dinnertime regardless of whether you are hungry or not.

- Eating because you won't have time or the chance to later on.

- Being told to finish everything on your plate as a child and you still do as an adult.

- Being told that you had to finish off your entire main course before touching your pudding.

Control

Take a quiet moment to reflect on your life and with a pen and notebook in hand, and ask yourself these questions and jot down your answers:

Is food the only part of my life I feel I have control over?

What does being in control mean to me?

In general, people who are healthily in control of their lives are not dependant on the reactions of others. They are not people pleasers. They would never do something that is against their own wishes just to stop their boyfriend / mother / husband from yelling at them / sulking / giving them the silent treatment. They do what is right and true for them without letting family members, friends or strangers manipulate them into doing something else.

They have a strong sense of self, of what their heart-felt desires are, and are happily involved in their own heart-felt desires. They are a joy to be around, and always have an encouraging word for those about them. Although sometimes thought of as selfish or unconventional, they are usually admired for their uniqueness. They are following their own inner directive, that still small voice within. When they do wish to change an aspect of their lives, or themselves, they usually do, because they are in control of their lives and themselves. They recognise a control freak when they see one, and do <u>not</u> let manipulative friends or family members affect them. They are generally positive folk, and we become more and more associated with them, and like them, as we give up compulsive eating.

By now you should have had some practice at trusting your body to tell you what it needs to eat, when to eat, and when to stop eating. You are trusting and following your hunger and fullness sensations, allowing them to be your guides while you are practicing being aware of and resolving those feelings that give you the urge to eat when full. So continue to move forward knowing that feeling your feelings is the bottom line alternative to binge eating because of them.

Hindsight – What to do after a binge?

There is naturally going to be some intermittent *eating when full* in the first few weeks and months of practicing the Am I hungry? assignment, until you are able to stop when full 100% of the time. Here is what to do when that overeating has occurred - Usually we feel riddled with guilt and self-loathing after a binge, but in truth, all is not lost. The more we can be understanding of, and compassionate towards, that compulsive part of our psyche, the better armed we are to overcome those compulsive tendencies. Here is what to do immediately after, or even a few days after a binge to still learn the valuable lesson of what caused it and how else it could have been dealt with:

What was the incident that caused the binge?

Example: *A stressful day at work and a fight with my husband.*

What feelings was I feeling about the incident?

Example: *Insecure and manipulated.*

How I dealt with those feelings and the incident?

Example: *I yelled at my husband and then binged on chocolate biscuits.*

How else could I have dealt with those feelings?

Example: *I could have gone to the bathroom when my husband started faultfinding. Breathed deeply and asked myself - Given the fact I feel this way what would I like to do now? – I might have got the idea to go for a walk to calm down and think.*

Many believe that you should only eat certain foods at certain times. The breakfast, lunch and dinner regime! No cereal in the afternoon please, and no garlic bread for breakfast! Please be relaxed and flexible, and even willing to be a little revolutionary (or evolutionary as I like to consider it) in your eating habits as you listen to your hunger and fullness sensations, and food fancyings. I remember being very surprised one morning when I distinctly wanted garlic bread! So, with a smile on my face I duly went about toasting some bread, spread my favourite vegan margarine on it, then spread on a crushed clove of garlic and a sprinkling of mixed herbs before popping it under the grill for another few seconds. You know, I thoroughly enjoyed that garlic bread for breakfast! It was just exactly what I fancied eating, when I was physically hungry, at eight am, that morning. And repeatedly women tell me this – how good, how really, really good, food tastes when it is the exact food they fancy eating, at that moment in time, when they are physically hungry. I later discovered that garlic is a natural antibiotic, so probably my body was helping me ward off a cold, or fight a mild infection of some sort through this particular food fancying. So do allow yourself ultimate freedom in terms of what you eat and when you eat for maximum benefit, bearing in mind our golden rule - be genuinely physically hungry when you eat. Your mealtimes may be a bit array, but you will be putting yourself in the position to lose any excess weight you might be carrying, for good.

Flexibility is the key here. If, for example you are hungry, at work and not allowed eat at your desk, this obviously makes things a little more difficult, but a small amount of nuts or dried fruit, a snack bar or chocolate bar, even a small sandwich in your handbag eaten discretely at some opportunity can often keep you going, and they don't take long to eat in these sorts of situations.

Women often ask me – What if I am preparing a meal for my husband coming home from work at 5 o'clock and I'm hungry at 4 o'clock? Do I eat then, and not eat with him?

What I suggest is this – If you are ravenous and can't possibly wait another hour to eat, you could have something small at 4 o'clock, whatever you fancy. That, you will find, will just take the edge off your hunger pangs and you could easily be hungry again when 5pm comes around and well able to eat something a little more substantial with your husband. As always, simply tune into your hunger and fullness sensations for ultimate guidance, and experiment with what you can do. Sometimes it works to just sit down with your husband while he eats, while you have a cup of tea. This is fine if you decide you want to eat something substantial earlier than he has his dinner. It is often just sitting together that is the important aspect of this.

So, let's not delay, if you are really hungry at 12 noon, know that it is ridiculous to wait until regimented mealtime at 2 o'clock before allowing yourself to eat. There is no point in causing yourself the needless discomfort of an empty stomach getting more and more empty, when you could be busily enjoying a tuna sandwich and cappuccino, at the local deli. Be kind and considerate to your stomach and yourself, when you are physically hungry, eat at that moment in time, without delay, and make sure it *is* what you really fancy eating, and stop when physically full.

A sense of control

In your ongoing journey of learning how to alter and change your eating patterns, to increase your sense of control around food, it is good to try leaving behind a spoonful or so, of each type of food, on your plate, at every meal. Simply leave it sitting on your plate and notice how you feel. Emotions and compulsive urges can be noticed and allowed to pass to reveal the underlying emotions. This practice helps you firmly establish a true sense of control around food, deleting the - 'I've got to finish off everything on my plate' - programming most of us received in childhood.

Leaving food on your plate can bring up uncomfortable memories of dysfunctional messages we got as children. Any of the following seem familiar?

'Finish, everything on your plate it is a waste to throw that food away.'

'After the time and effort I put into making that, and now you don't want to eat it!'

'Do you know how much that cost?'

'You cannot go out and play / leave the table / watch TV until you have finished everything on your plate.'

'Eat your greens they are good for you.'

'Look at all the starving in the world.'

'Finish your dinner and then you can have your desert.'

These statements did not take into account three very important considerations, in fact, these statements and ideas led you away from three very important considerations – Whether or not you were physically full, what you fancied eating, and what you fancied doing at the time. In other words you were robbed of your right to choose in the arenas of food and activity, and given false reasons for eating when full. Through this lack of choice, you were hindered in becoming fully self-determined. And when you think of it, what is life made up of except what and when we eat, and how we spend our time? That is it, that is life. Our childhood experience was of wanting to get up from the table when satisfied, to move on and do something else, and that got hindered by an adult saying (the words were slightly different but the message the same) - 'No, do not leave the table until you are stuffed.' We were quite literally ordered to eat when full. We were full, but had to eat – much the same feeling after a binge – Full, but had to eat. So, as children, the idea that *the body's own natural hunger and fullness mechanism cannot be true, and what mother says is true,* got firmly implanted in our young consciousness, even though mother's message was the ridiculous and fat-creating idea – *Do not stop eating when your stomach says you have had enough, keep stuffing in more food until I say you have had enough, or your plate says you have had enough by being empty.* So, as children when we were subjected to any, or all of the aforementioned ideas, we did not know what to believe, our own stomach's sensations, or what Mom was so adamantly stating. And we grew into women not able to trust our own hunger and fullness sensations that are still telling us, when to stop eating, and when to start eating.

Through no fault of our own, we learned to override our stomachs fullness sensations. So lets remember, the aforementioned statements lead to ideas of lack, limitation, scarcity and fear, which along with unresolved emotional issues are breeding grounds for addictions to flourish. These ideas learned in childhood and carried into adulthood, cloud *our relationship with food*, making it difficult for it to be the simple – I am hungry – I eat. I am full – I stop eating. Therefore, each of these statements needs to be questioned and undone, as they are not good enough reasons to eat when full and become overweight.

Heavenly State

Often I am asked – 'How on earth am I going to lose weight with my sweet tooth, and you telling me to eat whatever I want when I want, even if it is chocolate cake with coffee ice cream on the side for breakfast!?'

What a wonderful breakfast! And it is fine as long as you are **physically hungry,** for physical hunger is our gauge now. And the unhealthy aspect of all that sugar, cocoa and caffeine, well, as I mentioned before, *through allowance,* we learn we do not want to live off the stuff; it becomes, rather, a food we have when we fancy it, even if at strange times of the day. And through *the allowing of it, when we want it,* we do not tend to binge on it later. We know we can satisfy a little sugar or caffeine urge, as a wake-me-up, without guilt or it becoming a bad habit, a binge food, or a way to regularly suppress our feelings. Physical hunger, fancying, and moderation are the hallmarks of a healthy person's signal to eat. You are in the process of changing your relationship to food from an addicted one to a nurturing one, and you probably will binge / overeat intermittently (and as a result there may be some *temporary* weight gain) in the first few weeks of practicing your new ways of eating and relating to food and emotions. The real weight loss kicks in when you are stopping when full 100% of the time, not eating lettuce leaves 100% of the time.

Some weeks it will be 40% of the time stopping when full and 60% of the time various degrees of overeating. Other weeks it will be 90% stopping when full and 10% overeating. This happens because we cannot change ingrained habits overnight – it takes a bit of time, but it is time you have anyway, it is just *how are you going to spend that time?* You can spend that time overeating when the urge to do so arises, or you can spend your time noticing that you are full and addressing the emotions that are urging you to overeat. You can spend your time looking at, and resolving those emotions, following the healthy guidance you get as you ponder the much repeated, yet very important question – Given the fact I feel this way what would I like to do now? You can be forgiving of yourself, when the natural intermittent binge occurs, and simply pick yourself up, dust yourself down and get back on track with the **Am I hungry?** assignment until it is automatic.

You are now approaching your habit of eating when full from a new angle, and after a few binges you are even more aware of how physically uncomfortable binge eating / overeating really is. You are becoming more and more willing to feel the feelings that you used to binge to keep firmly under wraps. Overeating has already proven itself to be an inadequate means of coping, and you are now realising that you have a choice – Eat when full, suppress feelings, keep and gain excess weight, **or** stop when full, resolve feelings, lose weight and become slim.

Freedom and responsibility

In doing yourself the great favour of healing your own overeating habit, you are giving yourself freedom. Freedom from obsession, but remember awareness and responsibility are the price we all pay for freedom. Many people shy away from this word responsibility, but if you look closely, it is simply, the ability-to-respond. The ability-to-respond to life and what it presents you with in a way that enables you to live the life you want to live. After all, it is your life and only you can know what you want to be doing with it. Sometimes that is difficult to know, so we fall in with the norm when it is not satisfying to us, or we pander to the wishes of others rather than risk being the captain of our own ship. To begin the epic journey of your own life on your own terms, start asking yourself – What would I love to be doing with my time? Many people ask themselves this, and do this sort of daydreaming when they think about winning the lottery, feeling that large amounts of money alone, will give them permission to live life on their own terms. Money certainly helps, but you would be surprised how much you can accomplish on a shoestring, and I speak from personal experience. I have come to know that optimism, focusing on what you desire and taking step towards that, really can open doors in surprising ways. Yes the surprising reality of life is that many more dreams have been fulfilled by being focused and positive, employing persistence and creativity rather than relying on a huge lottery win. So even if we are not sure what we want in life, or we know what we desire, but never went for it because we simply did not believe it was possible, ceasing binge eating, and being more in-tune with, and able to deal with our feelings and emotional stuff, will play a big part in us being able to discover, move forward in the direction of our dreams, and make them a reality.

Food allergies

I have worked with many women who were on various restricted diets due to allergies. I have also encountered women who wish to abstain from certain foods, such as meat, dairy, sugar, chocolate and coffee. I myself, very happily, and easily, have not eaten meat or dairy for many years now, and a friend of mine had amazing health and energy while eating only raw. So let's look at this a little more closely: In my experience, simply saying to ourselves – 'Well I just won't eat that anymore,'- doesn't quite do the trick. Obviously more is involved, and more is required in order to successfully eliminate certain foods from one's food intake, and in taking a closer look at what is involved, I have discovered the following to be important keys, in the successful and continuous, happy, abstaining from specific foods.

Conscious awareness of what it does to your body – noticing any adverse reactions in your body every time you eat that particular food.

Permission to eat that which we wish to abstain from paradoxically opens up the choice to *willingly* refuse it.

Acknowledge it is not good for you because it causes adverse reactions in your body such as – Drink coffee, get a headache. Drink coffee, get jittery. Eat dairy – get blotchy skin.

Acknowledge that indulging in this food may be helping you distance yourself from certain feelings.

Intention to abstain from that food.

Willingness to abstain from that food.

Discovering the symbolic meaning of that food, by asking yourself: 'What is the essence of what I want here?' Example: Coffee equals romance. Cake is comfort.

Discovering other ways to bring that *essence* into your life. Example: I can ask myself how can I bring more romance into my life? I might go to Salsa or Tango class, as I love to dance. I can arrange a weekly night out with one of my friends to a local bar that plays live music.

Another example: I crave chocolate, but chocolate gives me migraines, so, I want to give it up, but when I ask myself – What does chocolate symbolise for me? I realise it symbolises *love and fun*. Therefore on a subconscious level, there is the conclusion - *If I give up chocolate, I give up love and fun.* So I ask myself – How can I get more *love and fun* into my life? What do I need to do to have more love and fun in my life? Or how can live without it more comfortably until it does come along? Well I can do the old-fashioned 'count my blessings' that always cheers me up. I can join a class I am interested in, people often go down the pub afterwards, and see if that livens things up a bit for me. I can watch a romantic comedy DVD or some of my favourite comedy shows. I can do some healing with a local healer, or NLP practitioner, on my emotional wounds that cause me sorrow.

Remind yourself why you want to abstain from this food you are allergic to.

Ask yourself What will abstaining from this food give me? More freedom? A greater sense of achievement? More energy? Less migraines?

Acceptance that you are ambivalent, at least some of the time, about giving up that food that you are allergic to.

Feeling any feelings of deprivation that come up when you choose not to eat it.

Asking yourself - Who am I allergic to? And feel the feeling associated with that person. Try doing 'The Work of Byron Katie' on that person (www.thework.com) Use the free Judge Your Neighbour worksheet, I have found it to be a fantastic, free, healing resource for issues with specific people.

We could be *allergic to* a judgemental parent, an alcoholic spouse, a relative we no longer see but they give us the creeps when we think about them. Often we need to learn how to deal with these people, understand them, see less of them or cut them out of our life completely.

Years ago, I made a friend at an evening class we attended weekly, and after a while I wanted to distance myself from her. Even though I liked her, I still felt allergic to her and her constant and persistent need for justification that always left me feeling drained. I began to realise her pattern – her common response to my stating how I felt about anything in casual conversation was always – Why? She was asking me to justify my feelings. This always took me aback, until I realised that it was her *learned way of responding* to someone having a feeling or preference. Something she was probably, subconsciously uncomfortable with because she never truly let herself feel her own feelings, or really acknowledge her own heart-felt preferences. Also, I realised that her parents probably responded to her in that way as a child if she expressed her feelings or preferences. In this way, her feelings were invalidated by the constant request for justification, implied in the word – Why?

She was simply, unconsciously, repeating a pattern of communication. I wondered how I could convey to my friend the message that the understanding of, and acceptance of thoughts and feelings, is more conducive to a contented life than the justification of thoughts and feelings. So, I would respond with a shrug of my shoulders saying 'I don't know. I just feel it.' Through this gesture I was able to stay centred around her, while conveying the message - 'It is not important *why* I feel it, it is important *that* I feel it.' I am not sure if I conveyed that message clearly, but I felt she was not open to any more analysis, and my job was not to change her, but to simply accept her, for I guessed her parents when alive rarely accepted her. I am off the judgement / justification roundabout. My dear friend was unfortunately still on it, and still suffering from the compulsion to suppress her feelings through eating when full. Her background of having had an alcoholic parent was still too painful for her to even acknowledge, she had a weight problem, and the judgement / justification game was still there, in her consciousness to be resolved.

And so, over the next few months I decided to stop attending that class as I was losing interest in the subject matter anyway and our friendship ended there.

Integrating feelings of 'missing out' when you abstain from the food you wish to give up.

Being still enough to observe yourself as you want or crave that food. Notice what thoughts come to mind and what feelings float through you as you, *be still,* and experience with a non-judgmental air of detachment, your own cravings and emotions.

If you do give in and eat it, do not beat yourself up about it, simply know that you are still reaching, in a dysfunctional way, for the meeting of some emotional need. If you indulge in that food when you are physically hungry, then at least you won't gain weight, you will just be suffering the adverse reactions that your body gives you as its means of telling you – *This food / beverage is not so good for me.* And an increased awareness of these adverse reactions, can serve, along with emotional resolving, to deter indulgence in that food the next time the urge to eat it occurs. When the next urge strikes, remind yourself – I can eat this if I want to, but do I *really* want to, considering how I felt the last time I ate it? And considering this food really means e.g. comfort, romance and fun to me, can I instead, go about really meeting those needs in real ways? What would that involve?

We have within us, the power to steer clear of food that we are allergic to, or simply do not want to eat, once we sort out the emotional stuff we have connected to that food.

I remember when I was pregnant my body giving me such definite signs as to what food I could and could not eat. So much so, that after two weeks I'd identified and abstained from the culprit foods that had my head in the sink. Throughout my pregnancy I successfully eliminated coffee, tea (except herb tea) cheese, milk, eggs, yogurt, butter, chocolate, sugar and pastries. If I had these foods at all, it was in very small amounts, and very rarely. And even though I had been vegetarian, I started to eat fish regularly, that, along with plenty of fresh fruit and veg., and a wonderful recipe for lentil pie, my 'in womb' baby and I thrived as a result of my listening to, and following, what my body was telling me. I was easily able to obey my body, because I had the above concepts, operating in my life.

But if you find it hard to break the habit of eating / bingeing on foods that cause you to feel bloated, hung-over, giving you a headache or a rash, then the way forward is to ask yourself – What was going on for me emotionally in the hours prior to indulging in that food? Once you realise *how you were feeling emotionally,* prior to your indulgence, then ask yourself – (like in the **What to do after a binge** assignment) *How else could I have dealt with that emotional stuff?* And use the answer as a guide as to what to do in future, when the urge to indulge in that food you are allergic to surfaces, which it will, for that is the nature of compulsions and unresolved emotional stuff – they just keep on surfacing again and again, until they are done and dusted properly.

In my opinion the true cause of a craving is always an unresolved emotional issue.

Suppressed emotions cause cravings, not the chemical reaction that the food induces. The chemical reaction that the food induces, such as the *sugar high or caffeine buzz* does not have the power to cause cravings in my opinion. I am not denying the fact that certain foods cause chemical reactions. Chocolate and sugar are well known for this. What I am saying is – the chemical reaction that particular food induces, is not the true cause of the cravings we feel towards that food. In other words, a sugar high does not have the power to trigger a binge, or make us eat sugar when we wish to abstain form it, but an unresolved emotional issue does. The cause of craving certain foods is always emotional. A craving can be described as the unconscious urge to put a feeling into suppression. A craving can be described as a yearning to meet, an unmet emotional need, in an inappropriate and ineffective way. A craving can be translated as a voice that says – Hey, there is a feeling coming into your conscious awareness that you do not like, a feeling associated with an unmet need, and your only known way of dealing with it, is to eat when full / eat that which gives you migraines / bad skin etc.

We will always be addicts if we feel the object of our addiction has any power over us. If we feel that one chocolate bar has the power to trigger us into eating three more when full, then we are giving our power away to a lie. The truth is, that within us, is a far greater power – the power that enables us to be free from addiction of any kind, the ability to stop after one chocolate bar, the ability to stop when full 100% of the time. The ability to abstain from meat, dairy, chocolate coffee, sugar and / or whatever we wish to abstain from.

True Slimness Weight Loss Principle # 12 Recognise and resolve the emotional issues that cause you to eat when full.

What is an emotional issue?

- That fight you had with your husband.

- The fact that you hate your job, are constantly irritated by your boss or can't stand the sight of your mother-in-law.

- That little incident with the shop assistant that left you upset and you don't know why.

- Your anger at your mother.

- Your non-existent relationship with your father.

- That friend that always leaves you feeling drained after talking with her on the phone.

- The fact that you have always wanted to join an art class but fear has always stopped you.

- You losing your temper big time, over little things.

- The need for more money.

- The need for more hugs and spontaneous affection in your marriage.

- The fact that when your husband comes home from work he stares at the TV screen for hours, and the conversation is zero.

These are emotional issues, and, as you realise by now, they are at the back of the urge to binge. An unresolved emotional issue is a challenge, a problem and a dilemma. So you see, true and lasting slimness, is all about what is going on in our hearts and minds, as well as what is going into our stomachs.

Resolving an emotional issue involves:

- Feeling feelings.

- Recognising and naming, if possible, your feelings.

- Thinking about how to solve the problem.

- Taking your focus of attention off the problem and on to the probable solutions.

- Letting go of the problem and acting on the solution.

- Dropping worry, going into trust and faith that the solution is appearing.

- Getting your emotional, physical and spiritual needs met.

- Asking our much-repeated golden question – Given the fact I feel this way what would I like to do now?

We are learning how to be aware of and observe, if you like, our emotions, realising that how we respond to our own emotions is important, rather than just blindly stuffing them down below our level of awareness with *food when full.*

Throughout this book I give suggestions as to what to do when feelings and emotional issues arise. One day when you are feeling sad you might find comfort in a good book or a favourite DVD, another day, when sad, you might feel drawn to phone a friend and suggest a night out to go dancing, and that will be the answer to the feeling of sadness. Another time it might be to pick up a favourite self-help book and doing one of the processes to tackle the root cause of your sadness will be the answer. The point I am making here is, that the solution is provided, only through your own *inner answers and gut feelings about what is right for you to do*, at any given moment in time, to help you deal with whatever feeling you are feeling.

All addictions serve the purpose of suppressing feelings.

Food addiction is eating when physically full.

True Slimness Weight Loss Principle # 13 Finding the way to resolve rather than suppress our feelings is part and parcel of healing addiction successfully.

What are you putting off doing until slim?

A sure sign of an unresolved emotional issue is when there is something that you keep putting off until you are slimmer. What are you telling yourself that you will do when you are slim? Make a list of all the things that you will not allow yourself to do now. It could be going out more, or swimming, or joining a dance class. The very fact that there are activities that you are putting off until you are slim, means you have half-hidden fears around doing those things. It is important that you discover what those fears are, and resolve them before you get slim. Otherwise you will get slim, and start doing a whole pile of things that you have unhealed fears about, this leads to anxiety and the tendency to binge due to these anxious feelings.

So, before you get slim, you can, for example, go to the swimming baths, and while there, *notice how you feel.* Believe me, if you feel vulnerable at the larger size you will not necessarily feel any less vulnerable a few sizes smaller. Body size alone, just does not have the power to banish vulnerability. Slim folk can feel just as vulnerable as larger folk. Now you can ponder how to tackle this issue of vulnerability, you can also decide whether or not you actually like to go swimming, maybe you prefer to go swimming in the sea with friends, to going swimming alone in a pool. Swimming feels the same fat or slim. It is just a sport, a leisure activity, and one of the many options of activities for you to incorporate into your life, regardless of your size or shape.

True Slimness Weight Loss Principle # 14 Start to incorporate into your life now, the things you think you will do slim.

You are learning how to overcome fears that stopped you from trying out something you thought you might like to do. It is as simple as that. We must remember that being slim in and of itself, cannot provide us with bags of extra confidence, or the ability, and permission, to do what we fancy doing. Only *you* can give *you* permission about what to do, and what not to do, in your life, regardless of your size and shape. It is a great shame to allow our body size dictate what we can and cannot spend our time doing.

Assignment

If you haven't done so already, make a list now, of all the things you think you will do when slim. I want you to look at your list daily, and seriously consider incorporating one or two of them into your life now. Consider what might be a little bit scary about doing those activities now, and seek to resolve those fears. What can you do to ease those fears? Are they rational or irrational? Choose one activity and bring it into your life by next week or as soon as possible.

We have a power point

That power point is the point when we are physically full and stop eating. From being physically full we can choose the healthy non-addicted, life-enhancing path of stopping when full. Or, we can choose the path of addiction, the self-defeating behaviour of eating even though we are full.

This is what happens at the power point: You have the compulsive part within yourself – that part of you that demands more food even though you are full. Please note that this compulsive part of you is only a part of you, and not all of you. You have other healthier parts and those parts are the ones we are bringing forth now in the recovery from compulsive eating. So open up a dialogue with this compulsive part of you, give her an age, picture her in your mind if you can, and have a chat with her. Do not scold her, be kind to her she is a wounded child, and, an unhealed aspect of yourself. I recommend Doris Cohen's web site www.drdoriscohen.com and her Seven Steps of Rebirth, another free resource for you to try from the smorgasbord of life tools, I suggest, as part of your healing journey.

Assignment

An encouraging thing for me to say to the compulsive part of me would be...

A reassuring thing for me to say to the compulsive part of me would be...

A forgiving thing for me to say to the compulsive part of me would be...

A loving thing for me to say to the compulsive part of me would be...

A respectful thing for me to say to the compulsive part of me would be....

An understanding thing for me to say to the compulsive part of me would be...

Positive self-talk is a form of giving yourself the love, attention, respect and acknowledgement that you did not receive (or did not receive in adequate amounts) as a child. This is what I call 'filing in the emotional gaps' - filling in those inner, empty spaces, left over from growing up that we carry with us into adulthood as unhealed wounds. These emotional gaps, which we all have to a greater or lesser extent, are the results of lack. Lack of love. Lack of approval. Lack of positive attention. Lack of reassurance. Lack of praise. Lack of harmony in the family or school. Lack of respect. Lack of hugs. This lack, this emotional vacuum, can be filled from within you, by you, when *you* give *you* understanding, reassurance, caring, time and attention. You giving to you. In truth, only when you are able to reassure, accept and approve of yourself, can you really begin to give it to, and receive it from, others.

Assignment

Ask yourself: If I were to receive acknowledgement and praise about something in my life, what would I like it to be for, and from whom?

Example: *I would like acknowledgement and praise for being a good mother from my husband.*

Now tell yourself (think it, or say aloud in private to yourself) – *You know what, you are a brilliant Mum!*

And notice what thoughts and feelings come to mind as you give yourself the words of acknowledgement and praise you long to hear. Do you welcome them? Does it feel uncomfortable? Any resentment that you may never hear them from the person you long to hear them from? Just notice the feelings and keep working with repeating the positive message until you can, indeed, take it on board and truly believe that message you are giving to you. Soon, you will see it in your life reflected in the eyes, words and actions of family and / or friends, strangers even. Your positive vibe cannot help but be reflected back to you throughout your life. You have filled in the emotional gap, healed a wound, chucked out and old, rotten, misery-creating belief and replaced it with a positive, life-affirming, nurturing one that ultimately brings out the best in yourself and others.

In this way you are learning to give yourself unconditional love, reassurance, praise and acceptance. Acceptance is so akin to love it is a vital component to health, wealth and happiness in my opinion, and if we did not get it growing up, then that is an emotional gap to be filled in by your own good self. Using the tips, tools, ideas, recommended reading and assignments in this book, you do find your way to the wholeness of a life without emotional gaps and compulsive eating. A life of true and lasting slimness.

Control

Many people fear *giving up controlling their food intake* and simply leaving that to their hunger and fullness sensations to dictate. It is an alien way to relate to food and eating for many, and a huge adjustment to make. Do you feel that food is the only area of your life that you have control over? If so, letting go of that last vestige of control in your life might be difficult. Trust is the answer we are looking for here. We replace *control* with *trust* – we are trusting our hunger and fullness sensations, and that innate wisdom of our bodies that I spoke about at the beginning of this book. So are you willing to let go? Yes, let go and trust! This is trusting your gut in more ways than one. Trusting it to tell you when you are hungry and full, and trusting it to tell you where to be going in life through your 'gut instinct' or intuition.

Cease Judging

Over the years in workshop after workshop, I have heard so many women discount their own feelings, calling them silly or stupid. Please, please, please cease judging a feeling as silly or stupid, for judging a feeling as silly or stupid is a sure way to put it into suppression. It is very hard to stay with, and experience a feeling, when you are busy criticising yourself for feeling that way in the first place. So do cease judging and criticising your feelings, rather say – *Ah that is interesting, so that is how I feel about so and so. Or, that is how I am feeling right now.* And then of course follow it up with - Given the fact I feel this way what would I like to do now?

Remember, you are <u>not</u> your feelings, you simply *experience* them. You are not your anger, fear or boredom. You are simply *experiencing the feeling* of anger, fear or boredom passing through you.

Become **the non-judgemental observer** of your own feelings.

Become **the non-judgemental observer** of your own thoughts.

Become **the non-judgemental observer** of your own compulsive behaviour.

For therein lies the power to change that behaviour. Awareness is the key in giving up any addiction and compulsive behaviour, be it eating when full, or anything else. Becoming more aware of how you think, feel, act and react, is the first step in transforming the self-defeating thoughts, feelings and actions into life-enhancing thoughts, feelings and actions.

Step by step this is how it looks – A quick summary:

1. You get slim by eating when physically hungry and stopping when physically full.

2. Stopping when full is made easier by resolving those emotional issues that cause you to overeat.

3. Resolving emotional issues is easier when you acknowledge your feelings and ask – Given the fact I feel this way what would I like to do now?

4. As you eat when physically hungry and stop when physically full your body automatically absorbs any excess fat cells. When there are no more excess fat cells, and as you continue to eat when physically hungry and stop when

physically full, your body maintains that weight loss effortlessly. Again both the absorption of excess weight and the maintaining of that weight loss occurs through eating when hungry and stopping when full.

5. You are happy with that result because of high self-acceptance, which we will talk about later in this book.

True Slimness Weight Loss Principle # 15 Don't judge your feelings, feel them. Feeling your feelings is the bottom line alternative to eating when full because of them.

The importance of being in touch with your feelings

It may seem like stating the obvious, but the following is true:

When you are in touch with your feelings, you know how you feel about Mr X and Ms Y.

When you are in touch with your feelings, you know how you feel about this situation and that situation.

When you are in touch with your feelings, you are in touch with life.

When you are in touch with your feelings, you are in touch with who you are.

It is a very dis-empowered state to not know how you feel about things such as your work, your boss, relationships, money etc.

When we are compulsive eaters, we might, quite literally, not know how we feel about certain things or people in our life. To a certain extent we are numb to the importance, or even existence of some issues in our life. Or, we may know how we feel, but are unable to act in accordance with those feelings. We may even deem those feelings unimportant or irrelevant. This is a very dis-empowered stance to take in life and not at all fulfilling. And it is a stance that we move away from, as we give up eating when full.

How we feel about things is extremely important, for it quite literally is valuable guidance and information that we need to learn to act on in effective and successful ways. If you are out of touch with your feelings you may not be in control of your life.

The ability to say – No – when you want to say no

- If you are unable to say 'no' in a situation where you want to say 'no' then you are not in control of yourself, or the part of the situation that you could influence – your part.

- If you are letting fear rule your life or even influence the decisions you make, making you act against your wishes, then you are not in control of yourself, or the part of the situation that you could influence – your part.

- If you do what other people want you to do, when it is against your wishes, you are not in control of yourself or the part of the situation that you could influence – your part.

If this is your experience of life, then it is natural to be feeling some uncomfortable feelings, such as fear, guilt, anger and sadness. And again, eating when full, will do little or nothing to help resolve this matter. Eating when full simply suppresses your feelings.

Maybe your uncomfortable feelings *are* telling you that you have little or no control in your life. These feelings, uncomfortable though they may be to experience – must be felt rather than suppressed in order for you to grow out of that situation and into a better one. The feeling of these feelings, the experiencing of these feelings, will help you alter the way you act and react to people and things, so that you are able to say – 'No' – when you do not want to do something. You can start being the person who, even if she feels afraid, still acts in accordance with her own heartfelt desires, and inner wisdom, of what is the best course of action to take in her own life.

It is indeed necessary for you to feel and acknowledge uncomfortable feelings, for feeling and acknowledging your feelings is the opposite of eating when full because of them. Acknowledge their message. Notice the unresolved emotional issue they are pointing to, that is crying out to be resolved, and ponder the solution to that issue, rather than running away from it through eating when full. Ask - What do I want from this situation and how do I go about creating that?

You are replacing *eating when full* with *feeling your feelings*. Know that by feeling it you are healing it – this is a gem of wisdom. Memorise it, and recall it often to reinforce within yourself of the value of *feeling,* emotions, rather than *suppressing* them by eating when physically full. This is what it takes to no longer binge eat – feel your feelings.

Use these affirmations upon waking to help keep you focused:

I intend to feel my feelings today.

I intend to resolve my emotional issues today.

I intend to only eat when physically hungry.

I intend to stop when full.

Intend to feel your feelings.

Be willing to feel your feelings.

Feel your feelings.

To suppress your feelings by eating when full, is suppressing or denying a part of yourself, and you cannot be whole and healthy with a part of you missing so to speak. When we feel our feelings, we are bringing back to ourselves the missing pieces, and becoming whole, and healthy, and slim.

A lot of the feelings we suppress are uncomfortable ones like anger, hate, jealousy or rage, and so it is understandable enough that we do not want to feel them. But emotions are always trying to tell us something, and these difficult ones are pointing to some lack of love, some injustice and some need not being met. Positive emotions like joy, peace, well-being and love, point out that we are on the right track in life, and that all is well.

When you deny your emotions, you are denying your very own self, and your own validity. You are invalidating yourself when you eat compulsively. Your very integrity is being invalidated and denied by you. Acknowledging is the opposite of denying. When you give up your addiction to *food when full,* by allowing yourself to experience those uncomfortable emotions, you quite literally start to validate yourself. You move into integrity. You begin to acknowledge, heal and / or communicate your feelings, deeming them important enough to be heard, first and foremost, by yourself.

What causes eating disorders?

Dysfunctional family background either mildly dysfunctional or severely so

Alcoholic parent(s)

Parent(s) with an eating disorder

Sexual abuse

Physical abuse

Emotional abuse

Overly critical parent(s) / teacher(s)

Emotionally distant parent(s) / teacher(s)

Bullying at school or from siblings

Any trauma (forgotten or remembered) that caused you to feel an extreme of emotion that you simply could not handle, so it automatically got repressed. The subconscious urge to keep it under wraps would cause you to eat when full.

It is important to realise that although these past dysfunctions do cause pain, sorrow and anger – they can only affect our lives negatively today, if we let them by continuing to eat when full because of them. In order to gain a positive 'now' out of the dysfunctions of the past, it is necessary to know that you have the power to stop suppressing your feelings, and can now start feeling your feelings, thus acknowledging and integrating them. Feelings are not wrong. It is appropriate to feel and experience anger, fear, rage etc when the past contained these instances of 'love absence'. We only get into trouble when we are frightened of our feelings, or judge them as silly or stupid, and eat when full to suppress them. Our feelings cannot control us unless we let them, we can choose which feelings to act on, and which feelings to *sit with* and simply allow to pass. What is important here is - You accepting your feelings, you developing the ability, through practice, to feel greater intensity of uncomfortable emotion without it driving you to the fridge when full. The appropriate expression and integration of these feelings, is your goal and your choice, in preference to suppressing your uncomfortable feelings.

True Slimness Weight Loss Principle # 16 Forgiveness empowers us to be the person to whom the dysfunctions of the past have no present day ill effect.

Forgiveness

Forgiveness does not condone the act we are forgiving. Forgiveness is claiming a divorce from past pain. Forgiveness does not mean we have to ever see the person we are forgiving again. Forgiveness gives us the freedom to live our best life, unhindered by the pain inflicted on us by others. Forgiveness is a *letting go* of that which no longer serves us well, in terms of emotion held in our own body, for when we hate someone, the emotion of hate is held in our own body, harming us, not the transgressor. Forgiveness empowers us to recognise and avoid abusers of all kinds. Forgiveness helps us protect ourselves, and our loved ones, for we are empowered to recognise and stay away from abuse of all kinds. True forgiveness is a relief, and a shedding of an old, tight skin.

Feeling and going through uncomfortable emotions

No one wants to feel bad. No one consciously wants to feel uncomfortable emotion. Most of us are not even that comfortable with seeing another human being feeling or expressing an uncomfortable emotion. As a whole, us humans, have together concluded that feelings in general are a bad idea, shaky ground and just plain weird, and if there is a distraction available, we'll take it. I see this going on around me in various ways, and to varying degrees of severity among young and old alike, as well as having experienced it played out in my own life. Oh what a circus! And what gets us to rethink all of that, is when the distractions do not work. The distraction of eating when full has left us fat. Now that is the biggest nudge isn't it? *Eating when full,* so as to *not feel bad,* causes such a huge side-effect that it cannot be ignored. The negative side effect of the dysfunctional coping mechanism of eating when full, literally clings to us 24/7! The coping mechanism isn't coping so good, in fact all it has done is left us with continued bad feelings, and excess weight to boot! That is when we search for an answer that points to the original culprit – What to do with this issue of *feeling bad*? And, when we are told – *Feel those feelings* - it is a bit like being told - *Well just continue to feel bad* – whatever that might entail, being bored, angry, hurt, resentful, out and out rage even, jealousy or fear. And again, none of us really want to do that. *But they pass,* I assure you. *Not very convincing,* I hear you say. Okay, but as I repeatedly state, actively seeking to *feel and resolve* the difficult or bad feelings of life, *is still and always will be,* the way out of all addiction.

Now, I understand that it is as if I am pointing you down a rocky road in order to get you to greater well-being, health and slimness. And I guess I am, but a rocky path can be incredibly beautiful, a road less travelled, not a monotonous highway. The rocky path will teach you awareness so you don't stub your toe. It has fine vistas, often giving way to peaks and valleys, and the beauty of this humble, rocky, path, can be magnificent at times.

Yet, if you choose the path of continued distraction, and suppression of feelings, you will end up stuffing your feelings down by eating when full, and carrying them with you, quite literally, for the rest of your days! Yes, that means all that stuffed down anger, is there contained in the fat cells of your body, all that suppressed grief, sorrow or frustration is in the very fat cells that cling to you, their host. An overweight woman carries around her emotional baggage 24/7. Does feeling feelings, seem, such a bad idea now?

☯

True Slimness Weight Loss Principle # 17 When I eat when full, I carry around my unresolved emotional issues 24/7 in the very fat cells of my body. When I feel my feelings, and resolve my emotional issues, I let them go for good. When I resolve my emotional issues, I no longer eat when full because of them, and I let the fat cells go for good.

Addiction is:

Addiction is anything that *momentarily* helps us feel better, but is, in truth, self-defeating behaviour.

Addiction always has a side-effect that eventually gets your attention.

Addiction is anything that distracts us from our feelings.

Addiction is a numbing of our feelings.

Addiction is *stuffing our feelings down* below our level of awareness.

Addiction distracts us from our feelings.

Addiction is anything that eases the pain *momentarily* by suppressing it, not resolving it, and in the long run, perpetuating it.

Addiction is anything that keeps us out of touch with our feelings.

Addiction is our old dysfunctional way of dealing with emotional issues, problems and uncomfortable feelings.

Addiction is what we are growing out of, and away from, by practicing its opposite – integration.

Integration is:

Integration is knowing how you feel at any giving moment in time.

Integration is being in tune with your feelings.

Integration is feeling, experiencing and acknowledging how you feel without judgment, criticism or blame.

Integration is making peace with a feeling, situation or trauma.

Integration is the resolving of a problem, dilemma, feeling or emotional issue.

Integration is being aware of and facing a problem, feeling or emotional issue.

Integration can result in bliss.

Integration is feeling good as a result of *the inner travelling through* an uncomfortable emotion.

All we have to do, to integrate a feeling, is, *feel it.*

Integration is our goal now.

Integration is the opposite of suppression.

True Slimness Weight Loss Principal # 18 Resolving emotional issues is the major healer of addiction. Natural abstinence from the object of addiction occurs in tandem with the resolving of the emotional issues that indulging in the addiction suppressed.

What's your question?

In order to be on top of your emotional stuff so that it does not get to crisis point, it is good to have a question about a particular issue that is unresolved in your life. Maybe a question concerning career or relationships.

Examples:

How can I find out more about a psychology course?

How can I meet more like-minded people?

How can I establish more joy in my life?

How can I heal the past?

How can I find out more about a career in teaching?

Resolving emotional issues – Assignment

Choose the area of your life that is the most important for you right now, and formulate a question, like in the aforementioned examples. Keep your questions in mind and be relaxed about it, knowing the answers are coming. Expect the guidance to come to you via your intuition. The thought to visit a friend you haven't seen in a while might occur, and when you visit her she mentions a book that you borrow from the library, and it happens to provide information that you need. A chance meeting at the local coffee shop might provide you with the information about an evening class that you are interested in. In this way we are actively *out there* meeting our own emotional needs, not binge eating because of them.

To deal with feelings ask yourself:

Yes, come back again and again to the old reliable - Given the fact I feel this way what would I like to do now?

To deal with life, relationships, work, love, money and spirituality, ask yourself:

How can I find out more about...? Fill in the blanks.

No more weights and measures

This means we give up weighing ourselves. Throw away the weighing scales if you can, or tape your ideal weight onto the little window on the scales. Why do this? Well, you know what happens when we weigh ourselves. Gain a few pounds, and we are down in the dumps. Lose a few pounds and we are elated. Stop allowing a piece of metal tell you whether to feel good or bad about yourself. Just resolve to feel good as you embark on the journey of stopping when full and resolving emotional issues. You will know you are losing weight because your clothes will tell you.

What makes a good day?

Example: *Going for a swim before work always puts me in a good mood, or doing a twenty-minute meditation upon waking.*

Resolve to do more of these activities that help you get the most out of life. Stop allowing weight loss be the only reason to feel good.

What makes a bad day?

Example: *Feeling invalidated by my mother when she phones.*

How can I deal with this problem so that I no longer eat when full because if it?

Example: *When I start to feel that feeling in the pit of my stomach, because she is talking over me, or not listening to me, I can make an excuse and end the call. A ten-minute conversation is usually enough for me if I am honest, and I am sure I can easily make sure the call does not last longer than that without offending her.*

Being in alignment

Chose an affirmation concerning an area of your life in which you wish to gain a specific result. This could be career, health, or finances. An affirmation is a positive statement, and always in the present tense. For example, for wanting to be slim, you state - 'I am slim.' Mentally repeat this statement and start to imagine it as true.

Picture that desired result. Close your eyes and actually see yourself slim, feel the feeling of being slim. It does not matter that your pictured results are very different to your 'now reality', it is just programming your mind to expect this as your, soon-to-be, reality. The visualised result is a message to your mind, that a healthier, slimmer you is a very real possibility now. It is *inner preparation* for the *outer result*. Also, any fears that come up can be worked through before you get slim, thus paving the way for lasting slimness. This is being in alignment – your desire, your thoughts, your pictures and your inner and outer preparation.

Compulsive eating the symptoms:

Thinking about food for a greater part of the day.

Having a love / hate relationship with food.

Being afraid of food.

Feeling powerless around food.

Eating compulsively – craving food when full – not being in control of your eating.

Being unable to stop eating when stomach is full of food.

Refusing to eat when hungry.

Thinking life would be better if slimmer.

When you start eating, being unable to stop, even when full.

Weighing yourself every day.

Not being able to leave food on your plate even though you are full.

Feeling guilty about wasting food.

Feeling guilty about overeating.

Not happy with, not accepting your size and shape.

Not in tune with the style of clothes you like. Instead, when at the larger size, you wear clothes to cover up your body, and when slim, you wear clothes to reveal your body.

What would it feel like?

Pick one issue that is your most pressing issue in your life? It could be your weight or your relationship with your spouse or child. And write down your most negative thought about that issue, and 'use a tool I mentioned before, 'The Work of Byron Katie,' author of Loving What Is. And on her website www.thework.com you will find a 'One belief at a time' download. And work on that negative thought.

You see, what I am doing is throwing tools at you. Tools to deal with your emotional issues that cause you to eat when full. I invite you to pick your favourites from these tools I suggest, so you can gather together your own personal tool kit that is your alternative to eating when full. Also ask yourself, concerning this issue: What would it feel like to have hope? What would it feel like to have faith that I am achieving my desired outcome? What would it feel like to have all my needs met in this area of my life?

We can be the person for whom the dysfunctions of the past have no present day ill effect.

I often joke with my clients saying - 'We all had a dysfunctional family!' I love to see their worried faces relax when they realise that it is not so unusual to have had a father who ignored and a mother who criticised or slapped. This does not condone that behaviour nor diminish the pain, it acknowledges the truth of the matter, in such a real way that it makes it something we *can deal with,* and no longer run away from. We realise we are not alone, and it wasn't our fault.

We are freed somewhat, to do the hard work, of undoing the negative present-day-effects of that ill treatment. And in so doing, we are also ensuring that our own children have a much happier, healthier childhood than we had.

What is suppression?

Suppression is <u>one</u> way of dealing with an unresolved emotional issue. It is <u>one</u> way of dealing with feelings that we are not comfortable with. It is a learned habit and can be unlearned. When we are compulsive eaters, eating when full, is our means by which we put a feeling into suppression. Life is gonna give us feelings, it is part of being human. What we do with those feelings is up to us, suppress or feel. Feeling is the healthy option, and if not learned in childhood, can be learned in adulthood, and this is what the real work of giving up an addiction, any addiction, is all about. It takes a lot of energy to put a feeling into suppression, and suppression loses it's appeal when we find another way of dealing with those same feelings, and emotional issues, that used to have us diving into the biscuit tin when full.

It is reassuring to know that there is no feeling that cannot be felt, or has not been felt, experienced and integrated by someone else before you.

This is subtle inner work and takes practice to master. Through turning your attention inward, you can quickly discover what is the best course of action to take at any given moment in time. If you allow yourself to recognise and trust this inner guidance, you can be accurately guided to the perfect outcome through your gut feelings, common sense, and intuition. The answers *are* all within you, and by asking the appropriate questions, such as those suggested in this book, you *can* uncover those priceless answers, and discover that acting on them is satisfying, life-enhancing and slim-friendly.

By now you are becoming more aware of when you are doing something to suppress your feelings, and you are practicing how to gradually bring in the healthy alternative. The repeated use of the healthy alternative that you discover from your continued practice of the 'Am I hungry?' assignment, is rapidly becoming your normal way of dealing with feelings and emotional issues that arise daily, in your life. You may already be finding that feeling and integrating your feelings instead of suppressing them, is a great relief, and very energising.

Emotions – a story from my own life

While working with a healer at one point in my life, I woke up early one morning finding the mood I was in and the emotions I was feeling, rather unpleasant, I thought – 'Oh no, I don't want to feel this way. I want to go back to sleep' (another avoidance tactic – sleeping too much). However, I knew that to get done what I wanted to do, I had to be up and awake, regardless of how I was feeling. So I got up, and in that early morning hour started to do my affirmations. As I did so I realised that an unresolved emotional issue was coming into my conscious awareness and I started to cry. I cried, and let myself feel the pain and sorrow of the issue until I felt it subside. I made myself a herb tea and went on with my affirmations. Then, with some time to spare before my baby would wake up, I started to work on this book and, as I sat in front of my computer, I discovered something I'd written some time before, and I instantly felt it to be the perfect piece of written material to add to the manuscript. As I beavered away I realised how much I love my work, and how the Universe always works with me when I open to its ways. I realised that my low mood had lifted. In fact my earlier sobbing had helped me clear out some old emotional stuff that I had been busily ignoring, and it had been dragging me down. Later that day, I was washing my French doors when I realised I was happy! *How true it is,* I thought, *emotions are just like clouds in the sky – they pass!* My uncomfortable morning emotions, had indeed passed because I'd had the courage to feel them.

Self-Acceptance

Self-acceptance does <u>not</u> mean that we have to stay the same weight.

Self-acceptance actually puts us in the position from which we are able to lose any excess weight permanently, and be happy with that result.

Self-acceptance is about taking responsibility.

Self-acceptance is about acknowledging with kindness, rather than judging.

Self-acceptance is the first step towards liking ourselves, and having healthy self-love.

Self-acceptance is empowering.

Self-acceptance is about taking the pressure off, and lightening up by saying – This is me, and I am okay.

Self-acceptance is facing up to the truth about yourself with kindness, forgiveness, love and understanding.

Self-acceptance is the seed that blossoms into self-confidence, self-esteem, self-worth, security and assertiveness.

Self-acceptance is the first step in becoming the person you want to be.

Again, both the absorption of any excess weight, and the maintaining of your slim body, is a direct result of eating when physically hungry and stopping when physically full, but happiness with that result comes as a direct result of self-acceptance, and *that*, we can develop now, at the larger size.

Self-acceptance is a commitment to <u>not</u> make a problem out of the self, whilst honouring a deep commitment to changing that which can be changed. You can change that which you wish you change about yourself. You can get to where you want to be without judgement. Criticising where you are, contrary to popular belief, does not make it easier to get to where you want to be. Criticising your size and shape does not make it easier to get slimmer. Self-acceptance and change go hand in hand. And acceptance is not *a resignation to the way things are,* but *an ignition of the power to transform the way things are, from within, out.*

True Slimness Weight Loss Principle # 19 Self-acceptance is a commitment to <u>not</u> make a problem out of the overweight-self.

How do I <u>not</u> make a problem out of, what clearly is, a problem, my overweight self? Well, it is a matter of perspective, getting into a perspective that will help you shed your overweight-self without giving it a hard time for simply, being, the result of you doing the best you could, at the time. It is the result of a dysfunctional solution (eating when full) and remember, we are changing our solutions from dysfunctional, to healthy and functional. And <u>not</u> beating yourself up for your size and shape, which is, after all, just the product of eating when full (which you are in the process of eliminating), empowers you to go about this difficult business of change. Changing your eating patterns, changing how you deal with your feelings and emotional issues. And ultimately changing your body size.

True Slimness Weight Loss Principle # 20 Self-acceptance is not about *resigning* to the way things are, but *an ignition* of the power to transform the way things are from within, out.

Ask yourself and several of your friends: Are you completely accepting of, and satisfied with, your size and shape? Prepare yourself for a few negative responses, even from your slimmer friends. The point I wish to make here is this – Most people are not at all accepting of, nor satisfied with, that which they have the most intimate connection to - their own bodies – the place they reside if you will. Changing this lack of self-acceptance, is one of the first three, most important steps, in healing your weight-gaining, eating habits, the other two being stopping when full, and resolving emotional issues.

Who would I be slim?

Write down, for every area of your life who you would be, slim, in that area. How would you react to your mother-in-law, for example, when slim? Would you be more assertive? More passive? Is your excess weight acting as a buffer between you and her? Who are you around your husband, when you are slim? More vivacious? Are you a woman getting a lot more attention from your husband now you are slim? Your work situation? How do you fit in, slim? Socially, out with friends or at the movies, swimming, on holiday, and with your kids? Is the slim you very different to the larger you?

Now, I'd like you to see how you can achieve those desired results, such as more assertive with your mother-in-law, now. Consider what it takes to bring in those changes in now, at your larger size, for a slim figure cannot do it for you, it has no power in and of itself, you give it power. It holds no guarantee of the positive results that you assume it will bring in its wake. These are issues that being slim has no influence over, and you will have to figure out the way forward, whether that is easy or difficult you will only find out as time passes, and you continue to use the processes in this book.

Suffering from compulsive eating and being overweight does not mean that you have to put your life on hold and feel diminished. In fact, a big part of the healing process as regards compulsive eating, is to pull the plug out, and get on with asking yourself - What would I *really love to do wear and be* – And get busy doing it, wearing it, and being it, regardless of your body size.

- We are no longer letting the fat stop us from doing what we want to do.

- We are no longer letting being overweight, be a reason not to be out there, living the life we want to live.

- We are no longer allowing excess weight be a valid excuse for not doing what we would love to do.

- We are no longer blaming our excess weight for certain problems in our lives, be it lack of love, money, friends, respect, contentment etc. We realise, we could have the exact same problem, slim.

True Slimness Weight Loss Principle # 21 Slimness is not the source of guaranteed happiness or anything else we might associate with it. It is, at best, only an influencing factor.

True Slimness Weight Loss Principle # 22 Discovering the source of happiness (or whatever desired quality you feel being slim carries in its wake) and practicing what it takes to become happy, is key, in permanent weight loss.

For me, I believe that being able to deal with what life gives you, brings happiness. Being able to resolve my emotional stuff, and heal my emotional wounds, through the ideas I talk about and mention in this book, has definitely been part and parcel of my own genuine, inner contentment that does not shirk downers, or bad hair days. The deep joy of knowing and following your own heart-felt desires brings an inner contentment that a slim body, alone, simply cannot deliver. Size and shape take care of themselves once we eat when hungry and stop when full, but inner bliss comes for dealing with the emotional stuff of our lives.

Being with people who leave us feeling good about ourselves helps, rather than spending time with people who criticise, ignore, or are rather negative in their outlook on life. Reading uplifting books, seeing uplifting films, watching great comedy shows like Seinfeld are all great ways to bring happiness. Being free from compulsive eating does bring relief and a greater sense of self, but you will not be promised a life without challenge, for challenge makes us grow, and is simply what we all have in life, but you will no longer be *eating when full* because of those challenges.

Owing our fat

Through the mind-frame of acceptance, instead of criticism towards our excess weight, we are owning our excess weight, and we have to *own something* before we can *lose it*. By increasing our self-acceptance, and really feeling a positive sense of owning our fat, we are putting ourselves in the position to lose that excess weight once and for all. We are saying that we are responsible for both the *keeping* and *losing* of that which we truly own. Not judging or criticising, not denying – owning. We spend so much time, either consciously or subconsciously denying our excess weight and feelings, deeming them ugly, and repulsive, something to be disguised or run away from, that we never take the time and effort, to simply be understanding of them. Rather like the mess a loving mother cleans up after her child, she knows it is not pleasant, but because she has love and understanding in her heart for her child, it is okay, she does it. A loving mother does not berate a sick child for throwing-up, she attends to the situation with love, genuine concern, efficiency and understanding. Be a loving mother to yourself, your feelings and your excess weight.

True Slimness Weight Loss Principle # 23 Self-acceptance and change go hand in hand.

Remember: Self-criticism only serves the purpose of keeping the old negative pattern in place, and the old negative pattern we are wanting to change here is – eating when full. Therefore when we actively develop our self-acceptance (which is the opposite of self-criticism) we are able to dislodge the old negative pattern of eating when full, and replace it, with the slimness-creating, and slimness-sustaining pattern, of stopping when full.

Fashion is fun

Develop the attitude that fashion is fun, and feel good about the clothes you wear regardless of how you think you pale in comparison to movie star magic, which usually involves a lot of make up and airbrushing. We are all divine daughters and sons of the Prime Creator of this glorious Universe. That force, that enables the stars to twinkle at night for our delight, that force that is the power behind the multiplication of cells which, in nine short months, becomes a complete and wondrous human being, that miraculous, little thought about force, is our mother – our loving mother, and we are, at the core of our being, as miraculous and glorious as She is, for She is within every cell of our being; otherwise we would not be living and breathing and walking around. So let's never consider ourselves as anything less than that fabulous truth about ourselves. To diminish or not recognise that truth is to shame ourselves, and deny our real self. Let your clothes and fashion take on their rightful role and be a joyous expression of your uniqueness. Let a world of ordinary, self-accepting goddesses and gods emerge of every size and shape, rather than a world of self-critical men and women, judgmental of their size and shape.

The idea that you are not going to wait until you are slim to wear the clothes you want to wear, or do the things you want to do, is a vital message for it touches on self worth. As compulsive eaters, somewhere along the way we decided to put our lives on hold. Almost as if we are going to be more worthy, more acceptable when slim. The truth is that you are acceptable and worthy and valid - right now. After all, giving up *food when full* is like an alcoholic giving up drink, and I definitely think to attempt giving up an addiction is highly commendable, and someone who embarks on *that*, is of great worth and highly inspirational to all around her.

True Slimness Weight Loss Principle # 24 I am a worthwhile person, whatever my size and shape. I am a good enough person whatever my size and shape.

Where does self-acceptance originate?

So, if self-acceptance is not an outcome of my size and shape, what is it an outcome of?

Self-acceptance develops within us in childhood as a direct result of good, caring, supportive parenting and tutoring. If you have low self-acceptance it can be attributed to how you were treated as a child and the conclusions you made about that treatment. Lack of parental approval, lack of emotional support, physical, emotional abuse are some of the contributing factors towards the low self-acceptance that a child could carry into adulthood. So, if these are the causes of low self-acceptance then simply changing your body size is going to do little or nothing to create high self-acceptance. The creation of high self-acceptance involves positive thinking and resolving the hurts of that upbringing.

True Slimness Weight Loss Principle # 25 Just as the creation of a slim body involves the ceasing of eating when full, along with resolving emotional issues, the creation of high self-acceptance involves positive thinking along with resolving emotional issues.

True Slimness Weight Loss Principle # 26 Resolving emotional issues supports a lot of positive change in our life. Resolving emotional issues is a very positive driving force – it allows positive change to be at the forefront of our lives in a very authentic and real way.

True Slimness Weight Loss Principle # 27 Self-acceptance is the climate through which the positive driving force of emotional resolving, travels, in its creation of positive change. Self-acceptance allows us to be contented with ourselves on the journey to slimness. Self-acceptance helps us welcome the arrival of slimness, and permanently live with the reality of being slim.

True Slimness Weight Loss Principle # 28 It is not about being in denial about your appearance or problems. It is not about beating yourself up about your appearance or problems. It is about taking responsibility for your appearance and problems in a non-judgemental way.

Lacking self-acceptance often causes us to look for acceptance and approval from others. This is actually a very dangerous thing to do, for in so doing, you can inadvertently sacrifice your needs, goals, beliefs and even your own heart-felt desires, not to mention the validation of your own feelings.

We are looking in the wrong place, when we look outside our own good self for acceptance. Self-acceptance cannot be found *outside*, it can only be developed from *within*. In thinking that you can gain a sense of acceptance by doing what another person wants you to do, instead of what you want to do, you sacrifice your life's purpose. In this way you give your power away. People who are manipulative or controlling are often addicted to control. Control is the object of *their* addiction. Our power effects the achievement of our goals. If we give our power away continually by doing something other that what we know is right for us to do, then we lessen the chances of our emotional needs being met, and we lessen the chances of achieving our own goals and heart-felt desires.

True Slimness Weight Loss Principle # 29 Addiction is a means of coping with a life that we are not yet satisfied with.

Through being more in tune with your feelings (as a direct result of stopping when full) comes the natural discovering of where life is taking us. This is what people call going with the flow. It is a tuning into a higher current that is providing us with everything we need along the way. Always in the direction of our likes, hopes and dreams, this going with the flow is another key to a happy existence. A life, and an existence in which you no longer binge.

Learning how to say – No – when you do not want to do something is a necessary challenge for the compulsive eating woman today. Not only saying – No – to food when you are physically full, but also saying – No – to whoever is asking you to do something you do not really want to do. For in so doing you are really saying a great, big - Yes - to yourself. Another key to happy, slimness-creating, living.

Asking for what you really want is big sister to the - *I can say no* – coin, and to know what you want (as mentioned previously) you have got to know how you *feel* about things. Hence the importance of acknowledging your feelings, experiencing your feelings, accepting your feelings, and faithfully behaving in a way that is in alignment with your heart-felt desires. In so doing *you* are acknowledging *you*. You are experiencing what it is like to be you. *You* are accepting *you*. You are being authentic. You are thus validating yourself and creating the life you desire. You know yourself and you accept yourself. Thus you become an empowered, genuine, dynamic (and slim) woman.

A change of focus

It is wise to want to be slim and healthy. To be slim and healthy is a goal all of us can certainly achieve but being obsessed with food and weight, is not necessarily part, of achieving it. We are changing our focus from obsession to health. We are changing our focus from *what it looks like,* to *what it feels like.* It does not matter so much *what I look like*, it matters much, much more *what I feel like, and how I feel.* You see the difference? Asking yourself – Am I sad, depressed, lonely? Or am I enlivened, joyous, content? What brings me those 'down' feelings? What activities, what people? Let me avoid them. What brings me those enlivened, *plugged-in to something good*, feelings? What activities, what people? Let me be around, and be involved with them. Am I helping me be out there doing what I need to do in order to be living the life that is right and satisfying, and true for me, bringing me the contentment and confidence I crave? Are the thoughts I hold, in the mind of my body, those of a confident, self-assured, self-accepting nature? Am I spending time changing my negative, self-defeating beliefs and thoughts into positive ones? These are the focus of your attention now. This is much more empowering than obsessing about outer appearance, and food.

True Slimness Weight Loss Principle # 30 How we look, is of secondary importance to the main issues in our life, which are what we think, and how we feel about things, these are of primary importance now, along with how we deal with those thoughts and feelings.

We take all that energy that we were putting into obsessing about size, shape, how we look and what we should and shouldn't be eating, and we channel it into considering how we are *feeling* and what we are *doing in life,* to help us be the fulfilled, contented, alive and vibrant human beings that we can be. High self-acceptance plays a big role in all of this. As you develop it through affirmations and the like, what you are doing is developing the inner knowing that:

What you say is important and valid.

What you do is important and valid.

What you feel is important and valid.

How you feel regularly now may be how you felt as a child

Good parenting ensures a child grows into an adult with plenty of confidence, happiness, security and other pleasant feelings about herself and the world in general. However, what parents and teachers often unknowingly do is undermine a child's natural self-confidence, or mar their happiness, or leave their children feeling insecure through inappropriate attention, or lack of attention.

We, as adults, may have forgotten the specific instances that caused us to feel unpleasant feelings such as self-consciousness, sadness and insecurity. But if you are experiencing these feelings on a regular basis in your present day life (or suppressing them by eating when full) – then it is more than likely that, *that* is how you felt at some stage in your childhood. It may have got repressed back then and you are feeling it now, in order for it to be resolved, forever. These old unresolved feelings, do indeed surface to be felt and healed. An uncomfortable, unresolved feeling in our awareness is asking for something, it is either pointing to an unmet need, in which case it is asking for the need to be met, or it is pointing to a negative thought or belief that is causing suffering.

True Slimness Weight Loss Principle # 31 By feeling your feelings you heal that which is causing you to eat when full.

☯

Tools of empowerment

Books: Books can be tools of empowerment, especially self-help books. The messages, information and ideas contained within their pages can be just what you need. So browsing the local library or bookstore shelves is often an extremely valuable use of your time. A book that provides the right information at the right time, is a wonderful blessing.

A new perspective: A positive thought, or *way of seeing,* is a tool. Suddenly a new thought comes to mind, a new way of looking at the situation that enables you to feel lighter and more resolved about it.

Affirmations: Affirmations are tools that enable us to change negative thoughts, beliefs and programs into positive, life-enhancing ones.

Visualisation: Visualisation is a tool to help us discover what is in the subconscious mind. Visualisation can help us uncover hidden fears that may block our progress. Visualisation can help us dissolve those blocks and visualisation can help us manifest our goals.

Anything that helps you feel your feelings: It could be a nice, hot, deep bath. It could be a walk in the park with your dog, a chat with a friend, a hug from your spouse, or a drive in the country. These everyday things are, in a very real sense, tools that can, quite literally, keep you afloat in the ocean of feelings that we sometimes feel we are at the mercy of.

A support group: I stress the word 'support'. Avoid any groups displaying signs of the 'poor me, ain't it awful,' syndrome. *That* will drain your energy and do little to help you feel empowered to overcome your habit of eating when full.

Natural therapies: From Rebirthing to Reflexology, Aromatherapy to Alexander Technique. From The Sedona Method to The Work of Byron Katie, from Bowen Technique to Bach Flower Remedies, natural therapies are healing aids and valuable resources for this business of learning, how to resolve, emotional issues that drive us, to food when full.

I can be the person who no longer turns to *food when full* to help her through.

☙

Assignment: Are any of the following familiar?

- Feelings that could be longstanding and recurring.

- Feelings that are so slight and small that you hardly notice them until a whole pile of them seem to have suddenly formed an emotional mountain that cannot possibly be ignored.

- Feelings that are positive, yet you find an underlying tendency to feel undeserving of the goodness of them.

- Negative feelings that are so familiar that you hardly know they are there. You take them for granted. Normal but negativity. *Doesn't everyone feel this way?* - you presume about these feelings.

Assignment: What's the message?

Every instance, feeling and situation has the potential to carry a message. So I would like you to, in a small notebook, jot down, over about a week or more, the various feelings, both positive and negative that 'come up' for you as your day progresses. And then, when you have a quiet moment, or at the end of your day, read through your list of feelings, and think about what message they may have had for you, as in the following examples:

1. *I felt pleased, happy and attractive when I got chatting to the man who sat beside me on the bus.*

2. *I felt annoyed with my boss for being aloof with me.*

What's the message?

1. *The message I get from feeling pleased and attractive when I spoke to the man on the bus is – I am ready to start dating again and 'You gotta get out more!' I feel, a desire to end my single status, was being highlighted by that chance meeting.*

2. *The message here is – Take the high road and send the boss universal love, and forgive her for being aloof. She has pushed your buttons because she really reminds you of your mother's aloof and cold behaviour towards you. So some forgiveness affirmations for Mum are in order. I also take it as a message to do that training course I saw on the Internet, and once I have that qualification, look for a position in another company.*

In the midst of feeling your feelings you can say the following to yourself:

- I accept this feeling completely now.

- It is safe for me to feel my feelings intensely.

- These feelings are passing through my being quickly and easily now.

Feelings are energy

Feelings are energy and energy can be blocked or free flowing. Suppressed energy is blocked energy, and blocked energy often manifests itself as physical pain such as a headache, or backache. See Louise L Hay's books You Can Heal Your Life and You Can Heal Your Body for information on how blocked feelings can be the root of disease, and how affirmations can heal. Blocked energy (blocked feelings) in the body not only can cause physical problems but also relationship or financial problems. Like water that ceases to flow and becomes stagnant, blocked energy causes blocks in your happiness, creativity, intuition, peace of mind, and fulfilment. Therefore we can know that our blocked or suppressed feelings greatly affect not only our weight, but our state of health. The solution is to allow all of your feelings to flow by feeling, or experiencing them. Flowing energy entails you acknowledging your feelings and taking them into consideration before you take action. Flowing energy is healthy energy. It gives you energy, good health and ideal weight.

The solution is to allow all of your feelings to flow by experiencing them, that means crying if you need to cry, beating pillows if you are angry. Thus you dissolve your energy blocks to achieving good, all-round, health.

Like an ever-changing symphony, feelings are an intricate part of being human. To flow with that symphony of life, learning better and better ways of handling your feelings is to be guided back to your real Self – the Self that can bring you the most out of life.

At the very core of your being, is a limitless fountain of love and bliss. Your essential nature is love. And a dynamic dynamo of positive energy to accomplish good lies at the very heart of *your* being, of every human being. Again and again the ancient and modern sages alike tell us this truth about our being. We get distracted from it through the hub-bub of day to day life. The pressures, the very real pressures of living, seemingly attack us and undermine our every attempt to be still and peaceful for even one moment. The world of Western culture seems to have little or no room for the beauty and grace of the realisation of our blissful, whole, nature, deep within. No medals for meditating on the divine within. Mockery can often be the reaction of any interest in the New Age or alternative fields. Distractions, lack of true understanding and support, threatens to keep humanity from discovering how to transcend the traps of suppressed emotions, and uncover a wonderful realisation – the bliss that is all-encompassing, the power to simply *be*.

Addictions and the stormy ocean of emotions, quite literally take our breath away, until we are breathing so shallowly that we cannot connect with how we *feel*. Distractions like movies, alcohol, and computer games, all compete for our attention, and offer quick fixes for the gnawing feeling that we are missing something really important here.

Maybe it is a major heart attack, a car accident, the death of a loved one, a divorce or financial crisis that causes us to look within, and ask the questions? 'What am I running from?' and 'What am I running towards?' The saying – 'There's got to be more to life than this!' – finally kicks in, and we do what it takes to discover the fundamental truth about who we are, and awaken to the beauty and grace of our authentic self, that lies beneath the surface agitation, of emotion.

As we start to unravel and resolve the complexity of our feeling nature, learning how to handle our feelings differently, we become more peaceful and less distracted from what is truly important. We realise, the true nature of being, is something that is a little closer to the divine than we ever, dared, imagine and that the inner world provides contentment and joy. Please encourage yourself to really experience and feel your feelings, allowing their energy to flow through you, for this is truly the secret to a happy, healthy life.

How many?

How many of us have lost weight only to regain it?

How many of us have lost weight only to fear putting it back on?

How many of us have lost weight with the gnawing anxiety of keeping it off, always with us, never really relaxing into the slimmer body size? How many of us have lost weight only to still be dissatisfied with ourselves?

How many of us have lost weight only to realise that we still have the same problems - problems we thought being slim would somehow help solve?

Maybe you are one of the many, many women who have had some or all of those experiences around weight. I know I have experienced *all of that,* over my five years, of compulsive eating.

Just think, *in reality,* how many people do *that* for the best part of their lives! And I really mean *best.* The best part of their lives, spent distracted from their feelings and to a certain extent, from their real inner knowing and strength, and from life. Time spent *waiting to be slim.* Time spent distracted from a true sense of self. The most tragic loss of all, is this loss of a truer, deeper, more meaningful *sense of Self.*

If there is any lesson in this, I believe it is this – To appreciate the seriousness of losing a few kilos or more – in no uncertain terms it is big emotional work, a date with the real you, ugly bits and all. The challenge of self-acceptance. The grace that stems from learning life's lessons, and the courage to face ourselves and our fears. The ability to be reborn through giving up an addiction, and allowing the true nature of your being unfold naturally. Acknowledging that oftentimes this is deep emotional work, may dishearten or even shock you, but let it not deter you from the task at hand, the ever present guidelines of a new, weight-loss, way of eating – stopping when full and resolving emotional stuff.

Life, life, what a precious gift that seems to get buried under a mountain of soap operas, work we do not really love, News bulletins, TV programs, house cleaning, family demands and necessary tasks, easy distractions and the many thoughts that hinder us from the *slowing down and inner connectedness* that encourages us to look at how we feel. It is a big deal to sit quietly when the kids are in bed, turn the TV off and let yourself feel your feelings, especially if they are as uncomfortable as having a sob and wailing – Why did my spouse leave? Why is life so hard? How can I deal with this? What is this pain inside? And how do I fill the emptiness that 100 cream cakes won't fill? So, I ask the all-important question again, how many people do you think go binge-eat because of this or similar emotional stuff, and have weight problems? I think we are talking millions. Some of them perfectly slim women, spending the majority of their time preoccupied with their weight, losing and regaining weight because they are too scared to ask the relevant questions to resolve these, or other emotional issues. Scared to seek and find an answer, scared to embark on the long, hard, haul until solutions of lasting, and real significance, and satisfaction come along, to help them heal and make the positive change from fat to slim.

Doesn't it shock you? It shocks me! What a waste! Perfectly beautiful, human beings, focused, obsessed and preoccupied with their weight. Through no fault of their own, wishing and hoping they were slimmer, instead of focusing on dealing with the very emotions that cause them to eat when full and thus gain weight.

I was one of those women, and the hope I offer you, is the reality I have given myself consistently over twenty years of slimness – The journey from fat to slim, the journey from compulsive eater to natural eater can be made.

☯

To be the very best we can be, to have our heart-felt desires come to us, is, strangely enough, often frightening. This relates to overeating, in that, often we are *eating when full* because we are not living the life of our dreams, or even acknowledging our heart-felt desires or giving them breathing space to manifest. We are not allowing ourselves the chance to grapple with the reality of success and failure. We binge because we are not in fulfilling work. We binge because we do not have any hobbies or interests that really absorb our attention. We binge because we have unfulfilling relationships and friendships. We binge because we are bored or stressed. We binge because we do not feel good about ourselves, instead of actively reminding ourselves of our good points and working on silencing that inner critic.

Being in tune with our own feelings, acknowledging and accepting who we are whilst working towards being the person we want to be, is a big section of the map that leads the way out of the addiction labyrinth. Be involved in what you love, ask yourself - How can I use what I have to get to where I want to be? And all the while, eat when hungry and stop when full, coming again and again back to our firm favourite concise and condensed formula as laid out in the **'Am I hungry?'** assignment at the beginning of this book. Let it be what you take away with you from this book, for it is, in truth, the whole course of what I teach, condensed. So imbibe it, allow it to be automatic and your new way of eating.

The moment is now, I am losing excess weight now

I am at ease feeling my feelings

Jealously is the feeling someone else has something (a material item, a relationship or quality such as beauty) that we desire for ourselves, and we feel we cannot attain that for ourselves. Reassuring yourself that you *can have what you desire* greatly helps ease jealousy. Of course you cannot *take* them from others, but the material items, relationships and qualities that you desire, are within your reach. A perfect equivalent of what another has, that is tailor made for you, can be on its way to you as you align yourself with your desires. Take comfort in the words of Abraham knowing they are true for you – 'There isn't anything I cannot do be or have and I have a huge Non-physical staff to assist me, and I am ready.'

Guilt is the feeling that I have done something wrong and the world is not a safe place. So really look at if you have done something wrong. And look closely at how you perceive the world. Do you perceive it as safe or friendly? Einstein has said that is the most important decision we could ever make. When we integrate our guilt we get innocence and strength and freedom.

Frustration has been described as diluted anger. When we feel our frustration it is always about limitations, so we can coolly look at our limitations and still see how we can overcome them, flow through, or round them like water, and have patience until things change if that is what is required. Integrated frustration is humility.

Assignment: Make a few brief notes about what from your family background could be affecting your eating habits today?

Example: *Mother always on a diet. Father being emotionally distant.*

Now for each answer I would like you to construct a forgiveness and release affirmation for the person(s) involved in these past events.

Example: *I forgive you and release you Mum. I forgive you and release you Dad.*

Write this affirmation out 15 times every day for about two weeks for this will help you contact and resolve the feelings you have around this person. You do not have to say anything to the person you are forgiving but you can if you wish to. By writing out the affirmation you are just quietly and purposefully cutting the unhealthy ties of hurt and / or anger that had bound you and this person together in an invisible, negative bond. Forgiveness dissolves that negative bond and heals you, frees you, and gives you more ability to draw to you the life you desire, the relationships you desire, and the weight you desire. Forgiveness helps clear away the emotional clutter within.

Now list three or more present day issues in your family that may be triggering the overeating. Example: *I work for my uncle and this work situation is definitely effecting my eating, it is so boring and tiring, I think I would feel guilty if I just up and left although I feel like doing that so often. The guilt causes me to binge.*

Now, I would like you to jot down possible and probable solutions to these present day problems. Steps that you could take, to make the situation more bearable, or help you move your life in a more fulfilling direction.

Example: *I could explain to my uncle how I feel and tell him I plan to look for another job, but will not leave until he has found a suitable replacement. Since guilt is often about feeling that we've done something wrong I could reassure myself I am doing nothing wrong in leaving this job. I could affirm 'Perfect employment is on it's way to me now, I could visualise my ideal job and hours. I could borrow some books from the library on the subjects I love, psychology and aromatherapy.*

True Slimness Weight Loss Principle # 32 The bottom line in healing addiction to food is feeling and integrating feelings we usually stuff down by eating when physically full.

True Slimness Weight Loss Principle # 33 The bottom line in natural permanent weight loss is to stop eating when physically full.

So, lets see how it is all connected. In order to be healthy we need to keep our energy or *chi* flowing, this involves experiencing our feelings, and, even if it feels a bit strange at first, experiencing feelings, is, I assure you, a most rewarding pursuit, and the basic tool of empowerment in giving up compulsive eating.

When we are busy feeling our feelings we are no longer suppressing them. As we are no longer suppressing them we are no longer blocking our energy through addiction. If we are not suppressing our feelings through eating when full, we are not doing that which is the cause of weight gain, and are allowing our body to lose that excess weight for good.

We are looking for and practicing that which enables us to feel our feelings and keep our energy or chi flowing. A pampering at the hairdressers when feelings of *failure* engulf you, instead of eating when full after work, for a week. The thought *I am good enough,* and actively choosing to believe it, when thoughts of a self-critical nature arise, instead of eating when full because of those negative thoughts, and the way they have left you feeling bad about yourself. A ten-minute nap when tired, instead of cake eaten when full with a mug of strong coffee when tired. The *issue* is the same. The *feeling* is the same. Tiredness is still tiredness. Failure is still failure. Self-critical thoughts are still self-critical thoughts that leave us feeling lousy. But your *way of dealing with them* is different. It is such a different way that it actually empowers you to make lasting changes in your life, specifically with regards to eating when full.

What is a treat besides food?

Example: *Ordering those rather obscure books I love from the library.*

Swimming in the sea.

Going to my local book club.

Pottering in the garden.

See if you can increase the amount of time you spend doing what you love, that way, food will not be your only treat in life. Food will be one of the many pleasures in your life but only eaten when genuinely physically hungry. And food when full, is even now, being easily given up as the old ineffective treat.

❧

Conjure up pleasant feelings

Feelings are like magnets that attract to them more of the same. It is a powerful tool to acknowledge that positive feelings can be conjured up from the very depths of our being. The pleasant feelings that you attribute to being slim are yours now, to summon up, no matter what size and shape you are. The seeds of these pleasant feelings may be dormant within you, but you have the ability to *feel them* with a little focused attention, imagination and a deleting of the negative thoughts that disagree with them, or would dampen them down.

Visualisation:

You can get a friend to read this aloud to you giving you a minute or two silence where there are dots - I'd like you to sit or lie down in a comfortable position and take a few deep, slow, breaths... Let your toes and feet relax, allow your calf muscles to relax... relax your hips and thighs... your stomach and lower back... relax you middle and upper back, your chest and shoulders... your arms and hands, feel yourself heavy in the chair as you let go. Relax your neck and jaw muscles; relax your facial muscles and your scalp... now do a quick scan of your body and notice if you are holding any remaining tension anywhere, and just release it, let it go... Good, now I'd like you to imagine a future imaginary event of your choice, at work or at home... at a party or wedding, and notice your surroundings... now imagine you feel the feeling you think being slim will give you... confidence for example. See yourself being this way... feeling this treasured feeling... and enjoying yourself in this environment... things working out well, things going in your favour... and now increase the good feeling you are feeling... make it feel really exuberant enjoy it... feel it and thus you embody it... Slowly let the scene fade and when you feel ready, open your eyes.

Thus you are familiarising yourself with what you desire e.g. more confidence. Remember being slim may enhance these feelings, but being

slim is not the source of these feelings. The source is deep within your being, and by practising conjuring up these positive feelings through visualisation you'll be able to draw on them when you need them in your day-to-day life.

Do remember the tools and ideas I give you are merely suggestions. Have no qualms about discarding some and embracing others as your own. And certainly develop the courage to seek out the books, groups and practices that will all combine together, to enable your own solution-finding-process, and ultimate healing.

I share with you the methods, tools and ideas that have enabled me to conquer the dysfunctions of my life. They can help you too. Your journey and healing is unique however. Where I choose rebirthing, you may choose Yoga. Where I meditate, you might have a reflexology treatment. I really think it does not matter. Your healing is in your hands, and what is important here, is that you actively and consciously seek it, enjoying the unfolding of your own individual path to well-being, allowing your inner knowing be your ultimate guide over and above all else.

More on feelings

If we can't name the feeling we are experiencing, we can focus on how we are feeling physically. We say things like – 'It was a gut wrenching feeling.' Or, 'I felt sick.' Or, 'My hands shook. I felt jittery.' All very physical sensations associated with intense feelings. If you cannot name the feeling that lies beneath your urge to eat when full, just describe it if you can. This helps you really acknowledge it as energy passing through you. Do not launch into self-condemnation if you find it difficult to describe or name how you are feeling, or are finding it difficult to find alternative ways of dealing with certain feelings. Some of this journey takes time, and the learning of skills as yet unknown. Some of this journey, of 'Discovering how to handle feelings,' *is* a real, trial and error experiment. Allow yourself time and space, along with loads of encouragement.

Please remember, as the coming weeks and months progress, our much repeated truth – eating when full suppresses feelings, but it is not the only way, and, in very subtle ways, we can suppress how we feel. Notice what other ways you might start to employ. Do you busy yourself with housework when your child needs your attention? Talk incessantly, never letting the other person get a word in edgeways for fear of actually noticing how uncomfortable you feel? These are more subtle ways of denying the task at hand, and avoiding how we feel. Unearth any compulsion in your behaviour. Simply notice it, and decide if it is what you want, and work on changing the behaviour you wish to change, and resolve any underlying emotional issues.

For example:

If you act distracted with your children, it may mean you can get on with the housework, but to meet their needs appropriately and cease cleaning and play snakes and ladders for half an hour (like they are asking you to do) may mean you feel, and integrate, some boredom. Or you realise for the first time, at a feeling level, the annoyance you feel towards your emotionally distant mother, who never had time to play when you were a child. You realise your mother was never really there for you. Thus, paying attention to your own children and breaking an automatic pattern of behaviour, you unearth and heal a chunk of your old, suppressed, emotional stuff. And when the kids are watching a DVD you can get on with the housework while thinking, 'I'll phone my friend with the twins, and invite her and the twins to come round for lunch and a play, because I have noticed, it is so much easier when my two year old and four year old have friends to play with.' A solution!

Life really can be this way – A problem, a solution. A problem, a solution. I'm hungry, I eat. I'm full, I stop eating.

Compulsive cleaning

When you've hovered up the Cocoa Pops for the fifteenth time that day, realise that you may be a bit obsessive about cleaning.

One woman told me – 'If my house was perfect then no one could fault me. At least that was under my control, even if nothing else seemed to be.'

These kinds of statements come up again and again. Women feeling that they have no control in their life. No power to really influence anyone or anything. Women have told me that they can only assert a voice in certain arenas, such as the food their children eat, the food they themselves eat, the clothes their children wear, the tidiness of their house. Maybe members of their family, their spouse or boss, either overtly or subtly overrules any decisions they have attempted to make, leaving them feeling powerless. Some women really do not have a voice. Their opinions are dismissed, not even considered by family, friends or spouse. And 'going it alone' may seem too daunting.

Rather extreme to think this can happen in this day and age, but nonetheless a reality for many. It is important to realise that if you are in such a situation, it will naturally cause you to feel feelings of an intense nature. These feelings are attempting to lead you out of that situation into a more nurturing one. *Intolerable feelings,* although uncomfortable, are *intolerable.* Their message is of vital importance to you fully realising the reality of your situation and the importance of you taking action to alter and change that situation.

True Slimness Weight Loss Principle # 34 Giving up eating when full always involves *a freeing up* of the avenues of expression – the throat and voice, avenues that can create positive change in our lives.

True Slimness Weight Loss Principle # 35 Giving up compulsive eating always involves looking at how we communicate with others.

Women who are stay-at-home wives and mothers often feel tied financially to their husbands. Even if they feel their marriage is over and they want to leave they are afraid to do so. Many women who are financially able to leave a relationship, are *emotionally not strong enough* to do so and thus are stuck in limiting circumstances. But the way forward is to simply keep alert for the next step, and it *will* present itself to you. It is trusting that there is a way to get to where you want to go, and you find it, one positive belief at a time.

By being willing to be responsible for *handling* our own feelings rather than just presuming that we are at the mercy of them, we are freer to give up compulsive eating, and we gain true self-control. This is a skill that in order to be mastered, requires the magic components of *knowledge, and intention,* along with *willingness to do things a little differently than before*:

- Acting and reacting to people in a more conscious manner.

- Sometimes saying things when you would have remained silent (and had a binge) before.

- Sometimes remaining silent or leaving the room when previously you would have stayed and shouted (felt guilty and overate) before.

Only you can know and implement what it takes to communicate who you are to the world about you. Only you can discover, by the trial and error method of experimentation, how to be, who you are.

Assignment

I would like you to imagine that you are already your slim-self and answer the following questions as if you are slim.

Are you happy?

Do you accept your size and shape completely?

Do you wear the clothes you want to wear?

Do you enjoy life?

Do you have a partner? If so, how is the relationship?

Do you like your body?

What job do you do?

How do you spend your free time?

Is there anything negative in your life?

Now comes the tricky bit

Look at your answers and either change your perception so that they would be true for you now at the weight you are now? In effect you are asking yourself what would, making that answer true now, or in the near future, involve? What steps little or big, would I have to take? What perspective about myself? What would I have to think and believe about myself, and my body, and my life?

Example: *When I answer – Do I like my body? As the slim me, the answer is automatically – yes. However at the moment, because I am larger than I'd like to be, my honest answer would be – no. In order for me to answer – yes, to that question now at the larger size I would have to develop self–acceptance, I would have to cease the self-criticising of my size and shape, and instead simply appreciate that my legs walk, my voice talks, my stomach is still able to tell me when I'm full, my arms can hug, my lungs breathe and my heart beats. Appreciation of the body because it works and I can still be kind towards it while developing a faith it will lose excess weight as I continue to stop when full. This will help me change my perspective to - 'Yes I like my body.'*

If you have completed that one I congratulate you! For it is one of the most difficult assignments to do – changing your perspective and facing up to what has to be done by you, now, in order to get the life you want and the figure you desire and deserve.

Put into practice the ideas that you have come up with in the second list, and watch yourself really accomplish your vision.

Slimness is just a body size

Happiness, self-esteem, confidence, love, beauty, success and contentment etc all come from within, through emotional resolving and positive thoughts, beliefs, words and actions, they can move to the outer, if they are not already a natural outcome of the parenting and tuition you received as a child.

True Slimness Weight Loss Principle # 36 Living the life you want comes from 'something other' than simply getting slim. Your job is to discover what that 'something other' is.

The point we are focusing on and learning here is that finding solutions to our problems comes from 'something other' than just being slim. Being happy comes from 'something other' than just being slim. Having a happy marriage comes from 'something other' than just being slim. Having a fulfilling career comes from 'something other' than just being slim. Like the cosmic carrot that the mystics tell us we follow from one good thing to another, in our constant quest throughout life, our job is to discover what that 'something other' is, whilst eating when hungry and stopping when full. That way slimness and solving problems occurs together.

Moving forward

With in the field of complementary medicine is the firm knowledge that the true key to well being lies in our own right relation to and understanding of, our very own feeling or emotional nature. In fact the exploration and understanding of emotions will no doubt be a usual class in schools and colleges of the future. This process has begun with pioneers like Brandon Bays' The journey, and The Work of Byron Katie already reaching schools, colleges and other educational and training institutions.

This is definitely not a matter of *getting rid of feelings* or suddenly having things easy. Life is about having emotions, and truly living is about having and solving our problems, or as I like to call them – challenges. If we would like to make life in any sense easier, then what we can do is work *with* the challenges rather than resisting, resenting or running away from them as we tend to do when we eat compulsively.

True Slimness Weight Loss Principle # 37 A big part of healing our eating habits and cease binge eating, is learning how to handle various fears that come up, as a natural part of living a full and active life.

Fear often arises when we think about or plan to do something new. Like enrolling in a night class or going for a better job, taking a step into the unknown, or taking a risk to attain a goal, and these are things we often have to do, in order to resolve, the emotional issues that cause us to eat when full. There is no way to be completely safe and certain all the time in a life that is truly lived. When we realise and accept this, we are really free to distinguish the snakes from the ropes on out life journey, and develop the ability to act accordingly. In the recommended reading section, there are many wonderful books, to aid the passage through and away from fear.

It has come to my attention, over the twenty years of being healed from my compulsive eating, that it has involved my being on a journey, a journey of healing to be sure, but also a journey of discovery, discovering who I am. And not only discovering who I am, but also unfolding and evolving who I am, in a sense, *expansion,* if you like. That journey has often led me inward, into my own feelings, my own consciousness, following what I love and enjoy, following my intuition or inner guidance. Doing what felt right and appropriate for me at the time, even though it might have sometimes seemed ridiculous, unwise, or unconventional to others, I realised that being 'true to my own nature' is an essential part of my no longer being a compulsive eater. No longer turning to food when full to help me through life, no longer suppressing my feelings, wants and heart-felt desires, meant no longer suppressing who I am, and who I am is so much more than being the slim, attractive woman.

I came to realise through my direct experience, that being who I am, is the key, not only to true slimness but also, the key to being whole, healed and healthy.

True Slimness Weight Loss Principle # 38 Much of giving up compulsive eating is about this core issue of being true to one's own nature.

True Slimness Weight Loss Principle # 39 Being true to ones own nature is easier when we accept ourselves, and if we work at raising our self-acceptance at the larger size, we simply bring it with us as we get slimmer.

True Slimness Weight Loss Principle # 40 When slim, you could meet the exact same challenges as you have now, or maybe different ones but meeting those challenges is all about setting boundaries.

Setting boundaries

Setting boundaries is an intricate part of natural permanent weight loss and facing fears and risking rejection is part and parcel of the fine art of setting boundaries. Many of us have never been taught to set boundaries, or have had our boundaries so disrespected that setting boundaries is totally alien to us. Well, all we need to do to remedy that is to know what our boundaries are in various situations, and when those situations arise, act in accordance with your boundaries. This is a natural outcome of knowing what you like, and want, and abiding by that. Acting in line with your own personal value system is a fine art and can be mastered over time. So, pursue a relationship if you desire. Take up meditation if that is what draws your attention. Do voluntary work if that is your calling.

Success

I love this quote by Ralph Waldo Emerson on success, he said that success is...

'To laugh often and much, to win the affection of children, to find the best in others, to endure the betrayal of false friends, to make the world a little better place to live in than when we were born into it, by rearing a little garden patch, improving some social condition, or helping a child grow healthier. To know that one life breathes easier since you lived. That is success.'

☯

A whole new way of eating evolves as we address our emotional issues in new ways – ways that no longer involve eating when physically full. The challenges of life do not necessarily disappear. What does disappear forever, is eating when full because of them.

And in meeting those challenges, the mystery of life is revealed and that mystery is here, as always, to be lived and enjoyed to the full.

☯

www.trueslimness.co.uk

Books:

Hiring the Heavens by Jean Slatter

Wishes Fulfilled by Dr Wayne Dyer

The Only Diet There Is by Sondra Ray

Why Weight by Geneen Roth

The Dynamic Laws of Prosperity, Catherine Ponder

Be Your Own Shaman by Deborah King

The Answer Is You by Michael Bernard Beckwith

One Day My Soul Just Opened Up by Iyanla Vanzant

Peace from Broken Pieces by Iyanla Vanzant

You Can Heal Your Life by Louise Hay

I Need Your Love, Is It True? By Byron Katie

Fat Is a Feminist Issue by Susie Orbach

Feel the Fear and Do It Anyway by Susan Jeffers

How to Stop Worrying and Start Living by Dale Carnigie

Women Who Love Too Much by Robin Norwood

Ask and It Is Given by Ester and Jerry Hicks

For further information about True Slimness workshops, phone sessions and individual consultations:

Email: sofia@trueslimness.co.uk

www.trueslimness.co.uk